CONTENTS

INTRODUCTION

The Innsky Air fryer is an easy way to cook delicious healthy meals. Rather than cooking the food in oil and hot fat that may affect your health, the machine uses rapid hot air to circulate around and cook meals. This allows the outside of your food to be crispy and ensures that the inside layers are cooked through.

The Innsky Air fryer allows us to cook almost everything and a lot of dishes. We can use the Innsky Air fryer for cooking Meat, vegetables, poultry, fruit, fish, and a wide variety of desserts. It is possible to prepare your entire meals, starting from appetizers to main courses and desserts. Not to mention, The Innsky Air fryer also allows homemade preserves or even delicious sweets and cakes.

How Does the Innsky Air fryer Works?

The technology of the Innsky Air fryer is very simple. Fried foods get their crunchy texture because hot oil heats foods quickly and evenly on their surface. Oil is an excellent heat conductor, which helps with fast and simultaneous cooking across all ingredients. For decades cooks have used convection ovens to mimic the effects of frying or cooking the whole surface of the food. But the air never circulates quickly enough to achieve that delicious surface crisp we all love in fried foods.

With this mechanism, the air is circulated on high degrees, up to 200° C, to "air fry" any food such as fish, chicken or chips, etc. This technology has changed the whole idea of cooking by reducing the fat up to 80% compared to old-fashioned deep fat frying.

The Innsky Air fryer cooking releases the heat through a heating element that cooks the food more healthily and appropriately. There's also an exhaust fan right above the cooking chamber, which provides the food required airflow. This way, food is cooked with constant heated air. This leads to the same heating temperature reaching every single part of the food that is being cooked. So, this is an only grill and the exhaust fan that is helping the Innsky Air fryer to boost air at a constantly high speed to cook healthy food with less fat.

The internal pressure increases the temperature that will then be controlled by the exhaust system. Exhaust fan also releases extra filtered air to cook the food in a much healthier way. The Innsky Air fryer has no odor at all, and it is absolutely harmless, making it user and environment-friendly.

Benefits of the Innsky Air Fryer:

•Healthier, oil-free meals
•It eliminates cooking odors through internal air filters
•Makes cleaning easier due to lack of oil grease
•The Innsky Air Fryer can bake, grill, roast and fry providing more options
•A safer method of cooking compared to deep frying with exposed hot oil
•Has the ability to set and leave, as most models and it includes a digital timer

The Innsky Air fryer is an all-in-one that allows cooking to be easy and quick. It also leads to a lot of possibilities once you get to know it. Once you learn the basics and become familiar with your Innsky Air fryer, you can feel free to experiment and modify the recipes in the way you prefer. You can prepare a vast number of dishes in the Innsky Air fryer, and you can adapt your favorite stove-top dish, so it becomes air fryer–friendly. It all boils down to variety and lots of options, right?

Cooking perfect and delicious as well as healthy meals has never been easier. You can see how this recipe collection proves itself.

Enjoy!

APPETIZERS AND SIDE DISHES

1. Japanese Tempura Bowl

Servings: 3
Cooking Time: 20 Minutes
Ingredients:

- 7 tablespoons whey protein isolate
- 1 teaspoon baking powder
- Kosher salt and ground black pepper, to taste
- 1/2 teaspoon paprika
- 1 teaspoon dashi granules
- 2 eggs
- 1 tablespoon mirin
- 3 tablespoons soda water
- 1 cup parmesan cheese, grated
- 1 onion, cut into rings
- 1 bell pepper
- 1 zucchini, cut into slices
- 3 asparagus spears
- 2 tablespoons olive oil

Directions:

1. In a shallow bowl, mix the whey protein isolate, baking powder, salt, black pepper, paprika, dashi granules, eggs, mirin, and soda water.
2. In another shallow bowl, place grated parmesan cheese.
3. Dip the vegetables in tempura batter; lastly, roll over parmesan cheese to coat evenly. Drizzle each piece with olive oil.
4. Cook in the preheated Air Fryer at 400 degrees F for 10 minutes, shaking the basket halfway through the cooking time. Work in batches until the vegetables are crispy and golden brown.

- **Nutrition Info:** 324 Calories; 12g Fat; 5g Carbs; 26g Protein; 9g Sugars; 2g Fiber

2. Mustard Cheddar Twists

Servings:4
Cooking Time: 45 Minutes
Ingredients:

- 2 cups cauliflower florets, steamed
- 1 egg
- 3 ½ oz oats
- 1 red onion, diced
- 1 tsp mustard
- 5 oz cheddar cheese
- Salt and black pepper to taste

Directions:

1. Place the oats in a food processor and pulse until they resemble breadcrumbs. Place the steamed florets in a cheesecloth and squeeze out the excess liquid.
2. Transfer to a large bowl. Add in the rest of the ingredients. Mix well. Take a little bit of the mixture and twist it into a straw.
3. Place on a lined baking tray and repeat with the rest of the mixture. Select AirFry function, adjust the temperature to 360 F, and press Start. Cook for 10 minutes, turn over and cook for an additional 10 minutes.

3. Sweet Carrot Puree

Servings: 4
Cooking Time: 5 Minutes
Ingredients:

- Salt, to taste
- 1 cup water
- 1 teaspoon brown sugar
- 1½ pounds carrots, peeled and chopped
- 1 tablespoon butter, softened
- 1 tablespoon honey

Directions:

1. Place the carrots in the Instant Pot, add the water, cover and cook for 4 minutes in the Manual setting.
2. Release the pressure naturally, drain the carrots and place them in a bowl.
3. Mix with an immersion blender, add the butter, salt and honey. Mix again, add the sugar on top and serve.

- **Nutrition Info:** Calories: 50, Fat: 1, Fiber: 3, Carbohydrate: 11, Proteins: 1

4. Healthy Parsnip Fries

Servings:3
Cooking Time: 20 Minutes
Ingredients:

- 4 large parsnips, sliced
- ¼ cup flour
- ¼ cup olive oil
- ¼ cup water

- A pinch of salt

Directions:

1. Preheat on AirFry function to 390 F. In a bowl, mix the flour, olive oil, water, and parsnip slices. Mix well and toss to coat.
2. Arrange the fries on the frying basket and place in the oven. Press Start and cook for 15 minutes. Serve with yogurt and garlic paste.

5. Baked Potatoes & Carrots

Servings: 2

Cooking Time: 40 Minutes

Ingredients:

- 1/2 lb potatoes, cut into 1-inch cubes
- 1/2 onion, diced
- 1/2 tsp Italian seasoning
- 1/4 tsp garlic powder
- 1/2 lb carrots, peeled & cut into chunks
- 1 tbsp olive oil
- Pepper
- Salt

Directions:

1. Fit the oven with the rack in position
2. In a large bowl, toss carrots, potatoes, garlic powder, Italian seasoning, oil, onion, pepper, and salt.
3. Transfer carrot potato in baking pan.
4. Set to bake at 400 F for 45 minutes. After 5 minutes place the baking pan in the preheated oven.
5. Serve and enjoy.

- **Nutrition Info:** Calories 201 Fat 7.5 g Carbohydrates 32 g Sugar 8.2 g Protein 3.2 g Cholesterol 1 mg

6. Cheese & Chive Scones

Servings: 10

Cooking Time: 10

Ingredients:

- 1 cup flour
- Salt and black pepper to taste
- ¾ oz butter, softened
- 1 tsp fresh chives, chopped
- 1 whole egg
- 1 tbsp milk
- 1 cup cheddar cheese, shredded

Directions:

1. Preheat on Air Fry function to 340 F. In a bowl, mix butter, flour, cheddar cheese, chives, milk, and egg to get a sticky dough. Dust a flat surface with flour. Roll the dough into small balls. Place the balls in the baking pan and cook for 20 minutes. Serve and enjoy!

7. Creamy Fennel(2)

Servings: 4

Cooking Time: 8 Minutes

Ingredients:

- 2 big fennel bulbs; sliced
- ½ cup coconut cream
- 2 tbsp. butter; melted
- Salt and black pepper to taste.

Directions:

1. In a pan that fits the air fryer, combine all the ingredients, toss, introduce in the machine and cook at 370°F for 12 minutes
2. Divide between plates and serve as a side dish.

- **Nutrition Info:** Calories: 151; Fat: 3g; Fiber: 2g; Carbs: 4g; Protein: 6g

8. Three Bean Medley

Servings: 4

Cooking Time: 15 Minutes

Ingredients:

- 4 cups water
- 1 cup garbanzo beans, soaked overnight and drained
- 1 cup cranberry beans, soaked overnight and drained
- 1½ cups green beans
- 1 garlic clove, peeled and crushed
- 1 bay leaf
- 1 small red onion, peeled and chopped
- 1 tablespoon sugar
- 2 celery stalks, chopped
- 1 bunch parsley, chopped
- Salt and ground black pepper, to taste
- 5 tablespoons apple cider vinegar
- 4 tablespoons extra virgin olive oil

Directions:

1. Place the water in the Instant Pot. Add the bay leaf, garlic and chickpeas. Also place the basket in the pan and add the cranberries.

2. Wrap the green beans in aluminum foil and place them in the steam basket. Cover the Instant Pot and cook in the Bean / Chili setting for 15 minutes.
3. Release the pressure naturally for 10 minutes, uncover the Instant Pot, drain the beans, discard them and place them all in a bowl. In another bowl, mix the onion with the vinegar and sugar, mix well and set aside for a few minutes.
4. Add the onion to the beans and mix well. Also add celery, olive oil, salt, pepper to taste and parsley, mix well, divide between plates and serve.

- **Nutrition Info:** Calories: 200, Fat: 1, Fiber: 6, Carbohydrate: 45, Proteins: 4

9. Sausage Balls With Cheese

Servings: 8
Cooking Time: 10 Minutes
Ingredients:

- 12 ounces (340 g) mild ground sausage
- 1½ cups baking mix
- 1 cup shredded mild Cheddar cheese
- 3 ounces (85 g) cream cheese, at room temperature
- 1 to 2 tablespoons olive oil

Directions:

1. Line the air fryer basket with parchment paper. Set aside.
2. Mix together the ground sausage, baking mix, Cheddar cheese, and cream cheese in a large bowl and stir to incorporate.
3. Divide the sausage mixture into 16 equal portions and roll them into 1-inch balls with your hands. Arrange the sausage balls on the parchment, leaving space between each ball. Brush the sausage balls with the olive oil.
4. Put the air fryer basket on the baking pan and slide into Rack Position 2, select Air Fry, set temperature to 325ºF (163ºC), and set time to 10 minutes.
5. Flip the balls halfway through the cooking time.
6. When cooking is complete, the balls should be firm and lightly browned on both sides. Remove from the oven to a plate and serve warm.

10. Simple Roasted Asparagus

Servings: 4
Cooking Time: 10 Minutes
Ingredients:

- 1 bunch asparagus
- 4 tablespoons olive oil
- Salt and pepper to taste

Directions:

1. Start by preheating toaster oven to 425°F.
2. Wash the asparagus and cut off the bottom inch.
3. Toss the asparagus in olive oil and lay flat on a baking sheet.
4. Sprinkle salt and pepper over asparagus.
5. Roast in the oven for 10 minutes.

- **Nutrition Info:** Calories: 127, Sodium: 1 mg, Dietary Fiber: 0.7 g, Total Fat: 14.0 g, Total Carbs: 1.3 g, Protein: 0.7 g.

11. Mac & Cheese Quiche With Greek Yogurt

Servings:4
Cooking Time: 30 Minutes
Ingredients:

- 8 tbsp leftover macaroni with cheese
- Extra cheddar cheese for serving
- Pastry as much needed for forming 4 shells
- Salt and black pepper to taste
- 1 tsp garlic puree
- 2 tbsp Greek yogurt
- 2 whole eggs
- 1 cup milk

Directions:

1. Preheat on AirFry function to 360 F. Roll the pastry to form 4 shells. Place them in a greased baking pan. In a bowl, mix leftover macaroni with cheese, yogurt, eggs, milk, and garlic.
2. Divide the mixture between the pastry shells. Top with the cheese evenly. Press Start and cook for 20 minutes. Serve chilled.

12. Kale Chips

Servings: 4
Cooking Time: 20 Minutes

Ingredients:

- 4 cups stemmed kale
- ½ tsp. salt
- 2 tsp. avocado oil

Directions:

1. Take a large bowl, toss kale in avocado oil and sprinkle with salt. Place into the air fryer basket.
2. Adjust the temperature to 400 Degrees F and set the timer for 5 minutes. Kale will be crispy when done. Serve immediately.

- **Nutrition Info:** Calories: 25; Protein: 0.5g; Fiber: 0.4g; Fat: 2.2g; Carbs: 1.1g

13. Feta Lime Corn

Servings: 2
Cooking Time: 20 Minutes

Ingredients:

- 2 ears of corn
- Juice of 2 small limes
- 2 tsp paprika
- 4 oz feta cheese, grated

Directions:

1. Preheat on Air Fry function to 370 F. Peel the corn and remove the silk. Place the corn in the baking pan and cook for 15 minutes. Squeeze the juice of 1 lime on top of each ear of corn. Top with feta cheese and serve.

14. Maple Shrimp With Coconut

Servings: 3
Cooking Time: 30 Minutes

Ingredients:

- 1 lb jumbo shrimp, peeled and deveined
- ¾ cup shredded coconut
- 1 tbsp maple syrup
- ½ cup breadcrumbs
- ⅓ cup cornstarch
- ½ cup milk

Directions:

1. Pour the cornstarch in a zipper bag, add shrimp, zip the bag up and shake vigorously to coat with the cornstarch. Mix the syrup and milk in a bowl and set aside.
2. In a separate bowl, mix the breadcrumbs and shredded coconut. Open the zipper bag and remove each shrimp while shaking off excess starch. Dip shrimp in the milk mixture and then in the crumb mixture while pressing loosely to trap enough crumbs and coconut.
3. Place in the basket without overcrowding and fit in the baking tray. Cook for 12 minutes at 350 F on Air Fry function, flipping once halfway through until golden brown. Serve warm.

15. Healthy Spinach Muffins

Servings: 12
Cooking Time: 15 Minutes

Ingredients:

- 10 eggs
- 2 cups spinach, chopped
- 1/2 tsp dried basil
- 1 1/2 cups parmesan cheese, grated
- 1/4 tsp garlic powder
- 1/4 tsp onion powder
- Salt

Directions:

1. Fit the oven with the rack in position
2. Spray 12-cups muffin tin with cooking spray and set aside.
3. In a large bowl, whisk eggs with basil, garlic powder, onion powder, and salt.
4. Add cheese and spinach and stir well.
5. Pour egg mixture into the prepared muffin tin.
6. Set to bake at 400 F for 20 minutes. After 5 minutes place muffin tin in the preheated oven.
7. Serve and enjoy.

- **Nutrition Info:** Calories 90 Fat 6.1 g Carbohydrates 0.9 g Sugar 0.3 g Protein 8.4 g Cholesterol 144 mg

16. Air Fry Garlic Baby Potatoes

Servings: 4
Cooking Time: 20 Minutes

Ingredients:

- 1 lb baby potatoes, cut into quarters
- 1/2 tsp granulated garlic
- 1 tbsp olive oil
- 1/2 tsp dried parsley
- 1/4 tsp salt

Directions:

1. Fit the oven with the rack in position 2.

2. In a mixing bowl, toss baby potatoes with oil, garlic, parsley, and salt.
3. Transfer potatoes in air fryer basket then place air fryer basket in baking pan.
4. Place a baking pan on the oven rack. Set to air fry at 350 F for 20 minutes.
5. Serve and enjoy.

- **Nutrition Info:** Calories 97 Fat 3.6 g Carbohydrates 14.4 g Sugar 0.1 g Protein 3 g Cholesterol 0 mg

17. Rosemary Chickpeas

Servings:4
Cooking Time: 20 Minutes
Ingredients:

- 2 (14.5-ounce) cans chickpeas, rinsed
- 2 tbsp olive oil
- 1 tsp dried rosemary
- ½ tsp dried thyme
- ¼ tsp dried sage
- ¼ tsp salt

Directions:

1. In a bowl, mix together chickpeas, oil, rosemary, thyme, sage, and salt. Transfer to a baking pan. Select Bake function, adjust the temperature to 380 F, and press Start. Cook for 15 minutes.

18. Green Mango Salad

Servings: 6
Cooking Time: 10 Minutes
Ingredients:

- 1/3 cup chopped cashews
- 2 mangos
- 1/3 cup chopped fresh coriander
- 1/3 cup chopped mint
- 2 tablespoons lime juice
- 4 teaspoons sugar
- 4 teaspoons fish sauce
- 1 tablespoon olive oil
- 1/4 teaspoon Asian chili sauce
- 1/4 teaspoon hot pepper sauce
- 1 sweet red pepper, thinly sliced
- 1 cup thinly sliced red onion

Directions:

1. Start by toasting cashews in toaster oven for 8 minutes.
2. Cut pointed ends off mangos, then skin.
3. Cut the mangos lengthwise into thin slices, then stack them on top of each other and cut again into thin strips.
4. In a large bowl, combine mint, coriander, lime juice, fish sauce, sugar, olive oil, and chili sauce.
5. Add mangos, red pepper, and onions to the bowl and toss.
6. Transfer salad to plates and sprinkle with cashews before serving.

- **Nutrition Info:** Calories: 140, Sodium: 317 mg, Dietary Fiber: 2.7 g, Total Fat: 6.2 g, Total Carbs: 20.7 g, Protein: 2.3 g.

19. Easy Crunchy Garlic Croutons

Servings: 4
Cooking Time: 20 Minutes
Ingredients:

- 2 cups bread, cubed
- 2 tbsp butter, melted
- Garlic salt and black pepper to taste

Directions:

1. In a bowl, toss the bread cubes with butter, garlic salt, and pepper until well-coated. Place the cubes in the Air Fryer basket and fit in the baking tray. Cook in the oven for 12 minutes at 380 F on Air Fry function or until golden brown and crispy.

20. Pineapple Pork Ribs

Servings: 4
Cooking Time: 30 Minutes
Ingredients:

- 2 lb cut spareribs
- 7 oz salad dressing
- 1 (5-oz) can pineapple juice
- 2 cups water
- Salt and black pepper to taste

Directions:

1. Preheat your to 390 F on Bake function. Sprinkle the ribs with salt and pepper and place them in a greased baking dish. Cook for 15 minutes. Prepare the sauce by combining the salad dressing and the pineapple juice. Serve the ribs drizzled with the sauce.

21. Healthy Barley Bread

Servings: 16
Cooking Time: 40 Minutes
Ingredients:

- 2 eggs
- 1/2 tsp baking soda
- 2 tbsp baking powder
- 3 cups barley flour
- 3 tbsp honey
- 1/3 cup olive oil
- 1 1/2 cups buttermilk
- 1 1/4 tsp salt

Directions:

1. Fit the oven with the rack in position
2. In a large bowl, mix together flour, baking powder, baking soda, and salt.
3. In a separate bowl, whisk eggs with honey, oil, and buttermilk.
4. Add egg mixture into the flour mixture and stir until just combined.
5. Pour batter into the greased loaf pan.
6. Set to bake at 350 F for 40 minutes. After 5 minutes place the loaf pan in the preheated oven.
7. Slice and serve.

- **Nutrition Info:** Calories 163 Fat 5.4 g Carbohydrates 26 g Sugar 4.6 g Protein 4.4 g Cholesterol 21 mg

22. Crispy Onion Rings With Buttermilk

Servings: 4
Cooking Time: 30 Minutes
Ingredients:

- 2 sweet onions
- 2 cups buttermilk
- 2 cups pancake mix
- 2 cups water
- 1 package cornbread mix
- 1 tsp salt

Directions:

1. Preheat on Air Fry function to 370 F. Slice the onions into rings. Combine the pancake mix with water. Line a baking sheet with parchment paper. Dip the rings in the cornbread mixture first, and then in the pancake batter.
2. Place the onion rings onto the greased basket and then into the baking tray. Cook for 8-12 minutes, flipping once until crispy. Serve with salsa rosa.

23. Salty Baked Almonds

Servings: 4
Cooking Time: 25 Minutes
Ingredients:

- 1 cup raw almonds
- 1 egg white, beaten
- ½ teaspoon coarse sea salt

Directions:

1. Spread the almonds in the baking pan in an even layer.
2. Slide the baking pan into Rack Position 1, select Convection Bake, set temperature to 350ºF (180ºC) and set time to 20 minutes.
3. When cooking is complete, the almonds should be lightly browned and fragrant. Remove from the oven.
4. Coat the almonds with the egg white and sprinkle with the salt. Return the pan to the oven.
5. Slide the baking pan into Rack Position 1, select Convection Bake, set temperature to 350ºF (180ºC) and set time to 5 minutes.
6. When cooking is complete, the almonds should be dried. Cool completely before serving.

24. Drunken Peas

Servings: 4
Cooking Time: 7 Minutes
Ingredients:

- 1 pound fresh peas
- 4 ounces smoked pancetta, chopped
- 1 green onion, sliced
- ¼ cup beer
- 1 tablespoon fresh mint, chopped
- 1 tablespoon butter
- Salt and ground black pepper, to taste
- 2 cups water

Directions:

1. Place the water in the instant jug, place the steam basket and set aside. In a heat-resistant skillet, mix the bacon with half the onion and spread over the bottom.

2. Heat on the stove over medium-high heat for 3 minutes, add beer, peas and salt, stir and remove from heat. Cover this pan with aluminum foil, place it in the steam basket, cover the Instant Pot and cook for 1 minute in the Manual setting.
3. Relieve the pressure, uncover the pan, add salt, pepper, mint and butter, mix, divide between the dishes and serve with the rest of the onion sprinkled on top.

- **Nutrition Info:** Calories: 134, Fat: 2, Fiber: 2.5, Carbohydrate: 10, Proteins: 4.3

25. Shrimp With Spices

Servings: 3
Cooking Time: 15 Minutes
Ingredients:

- ½ pound shrimp, deveined
- ½ tsp Cajun seasoning
- Salt and black pepper to taste
- 1 tbsp olive oil
- ¼ tsp paprika

Directions:

1. Preheat on Air Fry function to 390 F. In a bowl, mix paprika, salt, pepper, olive oil, and Cajun seasoning. Add in the shrimp and toss to coat. Transfer the prepared shrimp to the AirFryer basket and fit in the baking tray. Cook for 10-12 minutes, flipping halfway through.

26. Polenta Sticks

Servings: 4
Cooking Time: 6 Minutes
Ingredients:

- 1 tablespoon oil
- 2½ cups cooked polenta
- Salt, to taste
- ¼ cup Parmesan cheese

Directions:

1. Place the polenta in a lightly greased baking pan.
2. With a plastic wrap, cover and refrigerate for about 1 hour or until set.
3. Remove from the refrigerator and cut into desired sized slices.
4. Sprinkle with salt.
5. Press "Power Button" of Air Fry Oven and turn the dial to select the "Air Fry" mode.
6. Press the Time button and again turn the dial to set the cooking time to 6 minutes.
7. Now push the Temp button and rotate the dial to set the temperature at 350 degrees F.
8. Press "Start/Pause" button to start.
9. When the unit beeps to show that it is preheated, open the lid.
10. Arrange the pan over the "Wire Rack" and insert in the oven.
11. Top with cheese and serve.

- **Nutrition Info:** Calories 397 Total Fat 5.6g Saturated Fat 1.3 g Cholesterol 4mg Sodium 127 mg Total Carbs 76.2 g Fiber 2.5 g Sugar 1 g Protein 9.1 g

27. Blistered Shishito Peppers With Lime Juice

Servings:3
Cooking Time: 9 Minutes
Ingredients:

- ½ pound (227 g) shishito peppers, rinsed
- Cooking spray
- Sauce:
- 1 tablespoon tamari or shoyu
- 2 teaspoons fresh lime juice
- 2 large garlic cloves, minced

Directions:

1. Spritz the air fryer basket with cooking spray.
2. Place the shishito peppers in the basket and spritz them with cooking spray.
3. Put the air fryer basket on the baking pan and slide into Rack Position 2, select Roast, set temperature to 392ºF (200ºC), and set time to 9 minutes.
4. Meanwhile, whisk together all the ingredients for the sauce in a large bowl. Set aside.
5. After 3 minutes, remove from the oven. Flip the peppers and spritz them with cooking spray. Return to the oven and continue cooking.
6. After another 3 minutes, remove from the oven. Flip the peppers and spray with cooking spray. Return to the oven and continue roasting for 3 minutes more, or

until the peppers are blistered and nicely browned.

7. When cooking is complete, remove the peppers from the oven to the bowl of sauce. Toss to coat well and serve immediately.

28. Rice Broccoli Casserole

Servings: 8

Cooking Time: 40 Minutes

Ingredients:

- 2 cups brown rice, cooked
- 3 cups broccoli florets
- 1 tbsp olive oil
- 2 garlic cloves, minced
- 1 onion, chopped
- For sauce:
- 1 tbsp onion, chopped
- 1/4 cup nutritional yeast flakes
- 1 cup of water
- 1 garlic clove, minced
- 1 tbsp tapioca starch
- 1 cup cashews
- 1 1/2 tsp salt

Directions:

1. Fit the oven with the rack in position
2. For the sauce: add all sauce ingredients into the blender and blend until smooth.
3. Heat oil in a pan over medium-high heat.
4. Add garlic and onion and sauté until onion is softened.
5. Add broccoli and cook for a minute.
6. Add rice and sauce and stir to combine.
7. Transfer broccoli rice mixture into the greased casserole dish.
8. Set to bake at 400 F for 45 minutes. After 5 minutes place the casserole dish in the preheated oven.
9. Serve and enjoy.

- **Nutrition Info:** Calories 327 Fat 11.4 g Carbohydrates 49.2 g Sugar 2.1 g Protein 9.7 g Cholesterol 0 mg

29. Air Fried Eggplant Cubes

Servings: 2

Cooking Time: 12 Minutes

Ingredients:

- 1 eggplant, cut into cubes
- 1/4 tsp oregano
- 1 tbsp olive oil
- 1/2 tsp garlic powder

Directions:

1. Fit the oven with the rack in position 2.
2. Add all ingredients into the large bowl and toss well.
3. Transfer eggplant into in air fryer basket then places the air fryer basket in the baking pan.
4. Place a baking pan on the oven rack. Set to air fry at 390 F for 12 minutes.
5. Serve and enjoy.

- **Nutrition Info:** Calories 120 Fat 7.4 g Carbohydrates 14.1 g Sugar 7.1 g Protein 2.4 g Cholesterol 0 mg

30. Classic French Fries

Servings:6

Cooking Time: 35 Minutes

Ingredients:

- 6 medium russet potatoes
- 2 tbsp olive oil
- Salt to taste

Directions:

1. Preheat on AirFry function to 360 F. Cut potatoes into ¼ by 3-inch pieces. Drizzle oil on the potatoes and toss to coat. Place the potatoes in the frying basket and place in the oven. Press Start and cook for 20-25 minutes. Season with salt and pepper and serve.

31. Balsamic-glazed Carrots

Servings:3

Cooking Time: 18 Minutes

Ingredients:

- 3 medium-size carrots, cut into 2-inch × ½-inch sticks
- 1 tablespoon orange juice
- 2 teaspoons balsamic vinegar
- 1 teaspoon maple syrup
- 1 teaspoon avocado oil
- ½ teaspoon dried rosemary
- ¼ teaspoon sea salt
- ¼ teaspoon lemon zest

Directions:

1. Put the carrots in the baking pan and sprinkle with the orange juice, balsamic

vinegar, maple syrup, avocado oil, rosemary, sea salt, finished by the lemon zest. Toss well.

2. Slide the baking pan into Rack Position 2, select Roast, set temperature to 392ºF (200ºC), and set time to 18 minutes.
3. Stir the carrots several times during the cooking process.
4. When cooking is complete, the carrots should be nicely glazed and tender. Remove from the oven and serve hot.

32. Tasty Carrot Chips

Servings: 2
Cooking Time: 20 Minutes
Ingredients:

- 3 large carrots, washed and peeled
- Salt to taste

Directions:

1. Using a mandolin slicer, slice the carrots very thinly heightwise. Put the carrot strips in a bowl and season with salt. Grease the fryer basket lightly with cooking spray, and add the carrot strips. Fit in the baking tray and cook in the at 350 F for 10 minutes on Air Fry function, stirring once halfway through. Serve warm.

33. Pineapple And Cauliflower Rice

Servings: 6
Cooking Time: 20 Minutes
Ingredients:

- 2 cups rice
- 1 cauliflower, separated into florets and chopped
- 4 cups water
- ½ pineapple, peeled and chopped
- Salt and ground black pepper, to taste
- 2 teaspoons extra virgin olive oil

Directions:

1. In the Instant Pot, mix the rice with the pineapple, cauliflower, water, oil, salt and pepper, mix, cover and cook 2 minutes in manual mode.
2. Release the pressure naturally for 10 minutes, uncover the Instant Pot, mix with a fork, add more salt and pepper, divide between the plates and serve.

- **Nutrition Info:** Calories: 100, Fat: 2.7, Fiber: 2.9, Carbohydrate: 12, Proteins: 4.9

34. Baked Cauliflower & Mushrooms

Servings: 6
Cooking Time: 20 Minutes
Ingredients:

- 1 lb mushrooms, cleaned
- 8 garlic cloves, peeled
- 2 cups cherry tomatoes
- 2 cups cauliflower florets
- 1 tbsp fresh parsley, chopped
- 1 tbsp Italian seasoning
- 2 tbsp olive oil
- Pepper
- Salt

Directions:

1. Fit the oven with the rack in position
2. Add cauliflower, mushrooms, Italian seasoning, olive oil, garlic, cherry tomatoes, pepper, and salt into the mixing bowl and toss well.
3. Transfer cauliflower and mushroom mixture on a baking pan.
4. Set to bake at 400 F for 25 minutes. After 5 minutes place the baking pan in the preheated oven.
5. Garnish with parsley and serve.

- **Nutrition Info:** Calories 89 Fat 5.8 g Carbohydrates 8.2 g Sugar 3.9 g Protein 3.8 g Cholesterol 2 mg

35. Pineapple & Mozzarella Tortillas

Servings: 2
Cooking Time: 15 Minutes
Ingredients:

- 2 tortillas
- 8 ham slices
- 8 mozzarella slices
- 8 thin pineapple slices
- 2 tbsp tomato sauce
- ½ tsp dried parsley

Directions:

1. Preheat on Air Fry function to 330 F. Spread the tomato sauce onto the tortillas. Arrange 4 ham slices on each tortilla. Top the ham with the pineapple and sprinkle

with mozzarella and parsley. Cook for 10 minutes and enjoy.

36. Butterbeans With Feta & Bacon

Servings:2

Cooking Time: 20 Minutes

Ingredients:

- 1 (14 oz) can butter beans
- 1 tbsp fresh chives, chopped
- ½ cup feta cheese, crumbled
- Black pepper to taste
- 1 tsp olive oil
- 2 oz bacon, sliced

Directions:

1. Preheat on AirFry function to 340 F. Blitz beans, oil, and pepper in a small blender. Arrange bacon slices on the frying basket.
2. Top with chives and place in the oven. Press Start and cook for 12 minutes. Add feta to the bean mixture and stir. Serve bacon with the dip.

37. Paprika Potatoes

Servings: 4

Cooking Time: 30 Minutes

Ingredients:

- 1 lb baby potatoes, quartered
- 1/4 tsp rosemary, crushed
- 1/2 tsp thyme
- 2 tbsp paprika
- 2 tbsp coconut oil, melted
- 1 tbsp olive oil
- Pepper
- Salt

Directions:

1. Fit the oven with the rack in position
2. Place potatoes in a baking dish and sprinkle with paprika, rosemary, thyme, pepper, and salt.
3. Drizzle with oil and melted coconut oil.
4. Set to bake at 425 F for 35 minutes. After 5 minutes place the baking dish in the preheated oven.
5. Serve and enjoy.

- **Nutrition Info:** Calories 165 Fat 10.9 g Carbohydrates 16.2 g Sugar 0.4 g Protein 3.4 g Cholesterol 0 mg

38. Bok Choy Crisps

Servings: 2

Cooking Time: 10 Minutes

Ingredients:

- 2 tbsp olive oil
- 4 cups packed bok choy
- 1 tsp vegan seasoning
- 1 tbsp yeast flakes
- Sea salt, to taste

Directions:

1. In a bowl, mix oil, bok choy, yeast, and vegan seasoning. Dump the coated kale in the Air fryer basket. Set the temperature of your toaster oven to 360 F on Air Fry function and cook for 5 minutes. Shake after 3 minutes. Serve sprinkled with sea salt.

39. Savory Curly Potatoes

Servings: 2

Cooking Time: 20 Minutes

Ingredients:

- 2 potatoes, spiralized
- 1 tbsp extra-virgin olive oil
- Salt and black pepper to taste
- 1 tsp paprika

Directions:

1. Preheat on Air Fry function to 350 F. Place the potatoes in a bowl and coat with oil. Transfer them to the cooking basket and fit in the baking tray. Cook for 15 minutes, shaking once. Sprinkle with salt, pepper, and paprika and to serve.

BREAKFAST RECIPES

40. Lemon Vanilla Cupcakes With Yogurt Frost

Servings: 4
Cooking Time: 25 Minutes
Ingredients:

- Lemon Frosting:
- 1 cup natural yogurt
- 2 tbsp sugar
- 1 orange, juiced
- 1 tbsp orange zest
- 7 oz cream cheese, softened
- Cupcake:
- 2 lemons, seeded and quartered
- ½ cup flour + extra for basing
- ¼ tsp salt
- 2 tbsp sugar
- 1 tsp baking powder
- 1 tsp vanilla extract
- 2 eggs
- ½ cup butter, softened
- 2 tbsp milk

Directions:

1. In a bowl, add the yogurt and cream cheese. Mix until smooth. Add in the orange juice and zest; mix well. Gradually add the sugar while stirring until smooth. Make sure the frost is not runny. Set aside.
2. Place the lemon quarters in a food processor and process it until pureed. Add the flour, baking powder, butter, milk, eggs, vanilla extract, sugar, and salt. Process again until smooth.
3. Preheat on Bake function to 360 F. Flour the bottom of 8 cupcake cases and spoon the batter into the cases ¾ way up. Place them in the Air Fryer tray and bake for 8-12 minutes. Once ready, remove and let cool. Design the cupcakes with the frosting and serve.

41. Zucchini Breakfast Casserole

Servings: 8
Cooking Time: 50 Minutes
Ingredients:

- 12 eggs
- 2 small zucchinis, shredded
- 1 lb ground sausage
- 3 tomatoes, sliced
- 3 tbsp coconut flour
- 1/4 cup coconut milk
- 1/4 tsp pepper
- 1/2 tsp salt

Directions:

1. Fit the oven with the rack in position
2. Cook sausage in a pan until lightly brown.
3. Transfer sausage to a large mixing bowl.
4. Add coconut flour, milk, eggs, zucchini, pepper, and salt. Stir well.
5. Add eggs and whisk until well combined.
6. Pour bowl mixture into the greased casserole dish and top with tomato slices.
7. Set to bake at 350 F for 55 minutes, after 5 minutes, place the casserole dish in the oven.
8. Serve and enjoy.

- **Nutrition Info:** Calories 330 Fat 25 g Carbohydrates 5.7 g Sugar 2.7 g Protein 20.8 g Cholesterol 293 mg

42. Vanilla Granola

Servings:4
Cooking Time: 40 Minutes
Ingredients:

- 1 cup rolled oats
- 3 tablespoons maple syrup
- 1 tablespoon sunflower oil
- 1 tablespoon coconut sugar
- ¼ teaspoon vanilla
- ¼ teaspoon cinnamon
- ¼ teaspoon sea salt

Directions:

1. Mix together the oats, maple syrup, sunflower oil, coconut sugar, vanilla, cinnamon, and sea salt in a medium bowl and stir to combine. Transfer the mixture to the baking pan.
2. Slide the baking pan into Rack Position 1, select Convection Bake, set temperature to 248ºF (120ºC) and set time to 40 minutes.
3. Stir the granola four times during cooking.

4. When cooking is complete, the granola will be mostly dry and lightly browned.
5. Let the granola stand for 5 to 10 minutes before serving.

43. Spicy Apple Turnovers

Servings:4

Cooking Time: 20 Minutes

Ingredients:

- 1 cup diced apple
- 1 tablespoon brown sugar
- 1 teaspoon freshly squeezed lemon juice
- 1 teaspoon all-purpose flour, plus more for dusting
- ¼ teaspoon cinnamon
- ⅛ teaspoon allspice
- ½ package frozen puff pastry, thawed
- 1 large egg, beaten
- 2 teaspoons granulated sugar

Directions:

1. Whisk together the apple, brown sugar, lemon juice, flour, cinnamon and allspice in a medium bowl.
2. On a clean work surface, lightly dust with the flour and lay the puff pastry sheet. Using a rolling pin, gently roll the dough to smooth out the folds, seal any tears and form it into a square. Cut the dough into four squares.
3. Spoon a quarter of the apple mixture into the center of each puff pastry square and spread it evenly in a triangle shape over half the pastry, leaving a border of about ½ inch around the edges of the pastry. Fold the pastry diagonally over the filling to form triangles. With a fork, crimp the edges to seal them. Place the turnovers in the baking pan, spacing them evenly.
4. Cut two or three small slits in the top of each turnover. Brush with the egg. Sprinkle evenly with the granulated sugar.
5. Slide the baking pan into Rack Position 1, select Convection Bake, set temperature to 350ºF (180ºC) and set time to 20 minutes.
6. When cooking is complete, remove the pan from the oven. The turnovers should be golden brown and the filling bubbling. Let cool for about 10 minutes before serving.

44. Air Fried Philly Cheesesteaks

Servings:2

Cooking Time: 20 Minutes

Ingredients:

- 12 ounces (340 g) boneless rib-eye steak, sliced thinly
- ½ teaspoon Worcestershire sauce
- ½ teaspoon soy sauce
- Kosher salt and ground black pepper, to taste
- ½ green bell pepper, stemmed, deseeded, and thinly sliced
- ½ small onion, halved and thinly sliced
- 1 tablespoon vegetable oil
- 2 soft hoagie rolls, split three-fourths of the way through
- 1 tablespoon butter, softened
- 2 slices provolone cheese, halved

Directions:

1. Combine the steak, Worcestershire sauce, soy sauce, salt, and ground black pepper in a large bowl. Toss to coat well. Set aside.
2. Combine the bell pepper, onion, salt, ground black pepper, and vegetable oil in a separate bowl. Toss to coat the vegetables well.
3. Place the steak and vegetables in the air fryer basket.
4. Put the air fryer basket on the baking pan and slide into Rack Position 2, select Air Fry, set temperature to 400ºF (205ºC) and set time to 15 minutes.
5. When cooked, the steak will be browned and vegetables will be tender. Transfer them onto a plate. Set aside.
6. Brush the hoagie rolls with butter and place in the basket.
7. Select Toast and set time to 3 minutes. Return to the oven. When done, the rolls should be lightly browned.
8. Transfer the rolls to a clean work surface and divide the steak and vegetable mix between the rolls. Spread with cheese. Transfer the stuffed rolls to the basket.
9. Select Air Fry and set time to 2 minutes. Return to the oven. When done, the cheese should be melted.
10. Serve immediately.

45. Avocado Oil Gluten Free Banana Bread Recipe

Servings:x
Cooking Time:x
Ingredients:

- 1/2 cup Granulated Sugar
- 1 cup Mashed Banana
- 1/2 cup Light Brown Sugar
- 1/3 cup Avocado Oil, (or canola oil)
- 2 cups All-Purpose Gluten Free Flour, (see notes)
- 3/4 teaspoon Xanthan Gum, (omit if your flour blend contains it)
- 1 teaspoon Baking Powder
- 1/2 teaspoon Baking Soda
- 1/2 teaspoon Fine Sea Salt
- 2 large Eggs, room temperature
- 2/3 cup Milk, (dairy free or regular milk), room temperature
- 1 teaspoon Pure Vanilla Extract

Directions:

1. Preheat oven to 350°F and spray a 9x9 inch square pan with non-stick spray and line with parchment paper.
2. In a large bowl, whisk together the flour, xanthan gum, baking powder, baking soda, salt, and granulated sugar.
3. In a separate bowl, whisk together the mashed banana, brown sugar, oil, eggs, milk, and vanilla extract. Pour the wet ingredients into the dry ingredients and stir to combine.
4. Pour the batter into the prepared pan and bake at 350°F for 25-30 minutes or until a toothpick or cake tester comes out clean or with a few moist crumbs attached. Cooking time will vary depending on your oven - mine took 29 minutes.
5. Cool the bread in the pan on a cooling rack. Cut into 16 pieces and serve slightly warm or room temperature.
6. To store, wrap tightly in foil or store slices in an air-tight container. It will stay fresh up to 3 days. This bread also freezes well. To freeze, slice into individual pieces and freeze in a freezer bag.

46. Creamy Vanilla Berry Mini Pies

Servings: 4
Cooking Time: 20 Minutes
Ingredients:

- 4 pastry dough sheets
- 2 tbsp mashed strawberries
- 2 tbsp mashed raspberries
- ¼ tsp vanilla extract
- 2 cups cream cheese, softened
- 1 tbsp honey

Directions:

1. Preheat fryer on Bake function to 375 F. Divide the cream cheese between the dough sheets and spread it evenly. In a small bowl, combine the berries, honey, and vanilla. Spoon the mixture into the pastry sheets. Pinch the ends of the sheets to form puff. Place the puffs in a lined baking dish. Place the dish in the toaster oven and cook for 15 minutes. Serve chilled.

47. Bacon And Hot Dogs Omelet

Servings: 2
Cooking Time: 10 Minutes
Ingredients:

- 4 eggs
- 1 bacon slice, chopped
- 2 hot dogs, chopped
- 2 small onions, chopped
- 2 tablespoons milk
- Salt and black pepper, to taste

Directions:

1. Preheat the Air fryer to 325 ºF and grease an Air Fryer pan.
2. Whisk together eggs and stir in the remaining ingredients.
3. Stir well to combine and place in the Air fryer.
4. Cook for about 10 minutes and serve hot.

- **Nutrition Info:** Calories: 418 Cal Total Fat: 31.5 g Saturated Fat: 0 g Cholesterol: 0 mg Sodium: 1000 mg Total Carbs: 9.7 g Fiber: 0 g Sugar: 5.6 g Protein: 23.4 g

48. Breakfast Egg Tomato

Servings: 2
Cooking Time: 24 Minutes
Ingredients:

- 2 eggs
- 2 large fresh tomatoes 1 tsp fresh parsley Pepper
- Salt

Directions:

1. Preheat the air fryer to 325 F.
2. Cut off the top of a tomato and spoon out the tomato innards.
3. Break the egg in each tomato and place in air fryer basket and cook for 24 minutes.
4. Season with parsley, pepper, and salt.
5. Serve and enjoy.

- **Nutrition Info:** Calories 95 Fat 5 g Carbohydrates 7.5 g Sugar 5.1 g Protein 7 g Cholesterol 164 mg

49. Perfect Sausage-hash Brown Casserole

Servings: 12
Cooking Time: 45 Minutes
Ingredients:

- 6 eggs
- 16 oz frozen hash browns, defrosted
- 1/2 cup milk
- 2 cups cheddar cheese, shredded
- 1 lb breakfast sausage, browned
- 1/2 tsp pepper
- 1 tsp kosher salt

Directions:

1. Fit the oven with the rack in position
2. Layer hash browns in a greased 9*9-inch casserole dish.
3. Spread sausage on top of hash browns. Sprinkle cheese on top.
4. In a mixing bowl, whisk eggs with milk, pepper, and salt.
5. Pour egg mixture over hash brown mixture.
6. Set to bake at 350 F for 50 minutes. After 5 minutes place the casserole dish in the preheated oven.
7. Serve and enjoy.

- **Nutrition Info:** Calories 323 Fat 24.4 g Carbohydrates 11.7 g Sugar 0.7 g Protein 15.8 g Cholesterol 134 mg

50. Buttery Orange Toasts

Servings:6
Cooking Time: 15 Minutes
Ingredients:

- 12 bread slices
- ½ cup sugar
- 1 stick butter
- 1 ½ tbsp vanilla extract
- 1 ½ tbsp cinnamon
- 2 oranges, zested

Directions:

1. Mix butter, sugar, and vanilla extract and microwave the mixture for 30 seconds until it melts. Add in orange zest. Spread the mixture onto bread slices. Lay the bread slices on the cooking basket and cook in the oven for 5 minutes at 400 F on Toast function. Serve warm.

51. Breakfast Potatoes

Servings: 4
Cooking Time: 35 Minutes
Ingredients:

- 2 lbs potatoes, scrubbed and cut into 1/2-inch cubes
- 1 tsp garlic powder
- 1 tbsp olive oil
- 1/2 tsp sweet paprika
- Pepper
- Salt

Directions:

1. Fit the oven with the rack in position
2. Place potato cubes on the parchment-lined baking pan.
3. Drizzle with oil and season with paprika, garlic powder, pepper, and salt. Toss potatoes well.
4. Set to bake at 425 F for 40 minutes, after 5 minutes, place the baking pan in the oven.
5. Serve and enjoy.

- **Nutrition Info:** Calories 190 Fat 3.8 g Carbohydrates 36.3 g Sugar 2.8 g Protein 4 g Cholesterol 0 mg

52. Pea And Potato Samosas With Chutney

Servings: 16 Samosas
Cooking Time: 22 Minutes
Ingredients:

- Dough:

- 4 cups all-purpose flour, plus more for flouring the work surface
- ¼ cup plain yogurt
- ½ cup cold unsalted butter, cut into cubes
- 2 teaspoons kosher salt
- 1 cup ice water
- Filling:
- 2 tablespoons vegetable oil
- 1 onion, diced
- 1½ teaspoons coriander
- 1½ teaspoons cumin
- 1 clove garlic, minced
- 1 teaspoon turmeric
- 1 teaspoon kosher salt
- ½ cup peas, thawed if frozen
- 2 cups mashed potatoes
- 2 tablespoons yogurt
- Cooking spray
- Chutney:
- 1 cup mint leaves, lightly packed
- 2 cups cilantro leaves, lightly packed
- 1 green chile pepper, deseeded and minced
- ½ cup minced onion
- Juice of 1 lime
- 1 teaspoon granulated sugar
- 1 teaspoon kosher salt
- 2 tablespoons vegetable oil

Directions:

1. Put the flour, yogurt, butter, and salt in a food processor. Pulse to combine until grainy. Pour in the water and pulse until a smooth and firm dough forms.
2. Transfer the dough on a clean and lightly floured working surface. Knead the dough and shape it into a ball. Cut in half and flatten the halves into 2 discs. Wrap them in plastic and let sit in refrigerator until ready to use.
3. Meanwhile, make the filling: Heat the vegetable oil in a saucepan over medium heat.
4. Add the onion and sauté for 5 minutes or until lightly browned.
5. Add the coriander, cumin, garlic, turmeric, and salt and sauté for 2 minutes or until fragrant.
6. Add the peas, potatoes, and yogurt and stir to combine well. Turn off the heat and allow to cool.
7. Meanwhile, combine the ingredients for the chutney in a food processor. Pulse to mix well until glossy. Pour the chutney in a bowl and refrigerate until ready to use.
8. Make the samosas: Remove the dough discs from the refrigerator and cut each disc into 8 parts. Shape each part into a ball, then roll the ball into a 6-inch circle. Cut the circle in half and roll each half into a cone.
9. Scoop up 2 tablespoons of the filling into the cone, press the edges of the cone to seal and form into a triangle. Repeat with remaining dough and filling.
10. Spritz the air fryer basket with cooking spray. Arrange the samosas in the pan and spritz with cooking spray.
11. Put the air fryer basket on the baking pan and slide into Rack Position 2, select Air Fry, set temperature to 360ºF (182ºC) and set time to 15 minutes.
12. Flip the samosas halfway through the cooking time.
13. When cooked, the samosas will be golden brown and crispy.
14. Serve the samosas with the chutney.

53. Mushroom & Pepperoncini Omelet

Servings: 2

Cooking Time: 20 Minutes

Ingredients:

- 3 large eggs
- ¼ c milk
- Salt and ground black pepper, as required
- ½ cup cheddar cheese, shredded
- ¼ cup cooked mushrooms
- 3 pepperoncini peppers, sliced thinly
- ½ tablespoon scallion, sliced thinly

Directions:

1. In a bowl, add the eggs, milk, salt and black pepper and beat well.
2. Place the mixture into a greased baking pan.
3. Press "Power Button" of Air Fry Oven and turn the dial to select the "Air Bake" mode.
4. Press the Time button and again turn the dial to set the cooking time to 20 minutes.

5. Now push the Temp button and rotate the dial to set the temperature at 350 degrees F.
6. Press "Start/Pause" button to start.
7. When the unit beeps to show that it is preheated, open the lid.
8. Arrange pan over the "Wire Rack" and insert in the oven.
9. Cut into equal-sized wedges and serve hot.

- **Nutrition Info:** Calories 254 Total Fat 17.5 g Saturated Fat 8.7 g Cholesterol 311 mg Sodium 793 mg Total Carbs 7.3 g Fiber 0.1 g Sugar 3.8 g Protein 8.2 g

54. Crispy Crab And Cream Cheese Wontons

Servings:6 To 8
Cooking Time: 10 Minutes
Ingredients:

- 24 wonton wrappers, thawed if frozen
- Cooking spray
- Filling:
- 5 ounces (142 g) lump crabmeat, drained and patted dry
- 4 ounces (113 g) cream cheese, at room temperature
- 2 scallions, sliced
- 1½ teaspoons toasted sesame oil
- 1 teaspoon Worcestershire sauce
- Kosher salt and ground black pepper, to taste

Directions:

1. Spritz the air fryer basket with cooking spray.
2. In a medium-size bowl, place all the ingredients for the filling and stir until well mixed. Prepare a small bowl of water alongside.
3. On a clean work surface, lay the wonton wrappers. Scoop 1 teaspoon of the filling in the center of each wrapper. Wet the edges with a touch of water. Fold each wonton wrapper diagonally in half over the filling to form a triangle.
4. Arrange the wontons in the pan. Spritz the wontons with cooking spray.
5. Put the air fryer basket on the baking pan and slide into Rack Position 2, select Air Fry, set temperature to 350ºF (180ºC) and set time to 10 minutes.
6. Flip the wontons halfway through the cooking time.
7. When cooking is complete, the wontons will be crispy and golden brown.
8. Serve immediately.

55. Cheesy Baked-egg Toast

Servings: 4
Cooking Time: 10 Minutes
Ingredients:

- 4 slices wheat bread
- 4 eggs
- 1 cup shredded cheese
- 2 tablespoons softened butter

Directions:

1. Start by preheating toaster oven to 350°F.
2. Place bread on a greased baking sheet.
3. Use a teaspoon to push a square into the bread creating a little bed for the egg.
4. Sprinkle salt and pepper over the bread.
5. Break one egg into each square. Spread butter over each edge of the bread.
6. Sprinkle 1/4 cup cheese over buttered area.
7. Bake for 10 minutes or until the eggs are solid and the cheese is golden brown.

- **Nutrition Info:** Calories: 297, Sodium: 410 mg, Dietary Fiber: 1.9 g, Total Fat: 20.4 g, Total Carbs: 12.3 g, Protein: 16.3 g.

56. Hashbrown Breakfast Casserole

Servings: 8
Cooking Time: 50 Minutes
Ingredients:

- 3 cups shredded cauliflower
- 1/2 cup mayonnaise
- 1 cup sour cream
- 4 tbsp butter
- 1 tbsp bouillon powder
- 1 tbsp onion, minced
- 1 cup cheddar cheese, shredded
- 1/2 tsp pepper
- 1 tsp salt

Directions:

1. Fit the oven with the rack in position
2. Set aside 1/3 cup shredded cheese.

3. In a bowl, add remaining ingredients and mix well.
4. Spread mixture into the greased 8*8-inch baking dish and sprinkle with remaining shredded cheese.
5. Set to bake at 350 F for 55 minutes. After 5 minutes place the baking dish in the preheated oven.
6. Serve and enjoy.

- **Nutrition Info:** Calories 237 Fat 21.4 g Carbohydrates 7.1 g Sugar 2 g Protein 5.4 g Cholesterol 47 mg

57. Latkes

Servings: 5
Cooking Time: 7 Minutes
Ingredients:

- 1 large onion
- 5 large potatoes peeled
- 4 large eggs
- ¼ cup potato starch
- 2 tsp kosher salt
- ½ tsp baking powder
- Olive oil

Directions:

1. Scrub your potatoes well and place them in a food processor. Besides, place the shredded potatoes in a bowl of cool water and set it aside.
2. Rinse the food in the processor and grate the onions. Place your grated onions in a paper towel and squeeze out the liquid.
3. In a medium sized bowl whisk your eggs and add matzo, pepper, 1 tsp potato starch, baking powder and grated onion. Drain the water from the potatoes and save the starch that remains in your bowl.
4. Scoop the starch from the potato bowl and add to the latke mixture. Form latkes from the mixture in flat circles and dip into dry potato starch. Add oil and place them in an air fryer
5. Air fry your latkes at 360-degree Fahrenheit for 8 minutes
6. and turn in the middle once it indicates turn food.
7. Serve while hot.

- **Nutrition Info:** Calories 68 Fat 4g, Carbohydrates 6g, Protein 2g.

58. Vanilla & Cinnamon Toast Toppet

Servings: 6
Cooking Time: 10 Minutes
Ingredients:

- 12 slices bread
- ½ cup sugar
- 1 ½ tsp cinnamon
- 1 stick of butter, softened
- 1 tsp vanilla extract

Directions:

1. Preheat on Toast function to 360 F. Combine all ingredients, except the bread, in a bowl. Spread the buttery cinnamon mixture onto the bread slices. Place the bread slices in the toaster oven. Cook for 8 minutes. Serve.

59. Crispy Cauliflowers With Alfredo Sauce

Servings:4
Cooking Time: 20 Minutes
Ingredients:

- 4 cups cauliflower florets
- 1 tbsp butter, melted
- ¼ cup alfredo sauce
- 1 cup breadcrumbs
- 1 tsp salt

Directions:

1. Whisk alfredo sauce with butter. In a bowl, combine breadcrumbs with salt. Dip cauliflower into the alfredo mixture and then coat in the crumbs. Drop the prepared florets into the frying basket. Set the temperature to 350 F and press Start. Cook for 15 minutes on AirFry function.

60. Caprese Sourdough Sandwich

Servings:2
Cooking Time: 25 Minutes
Ingredients:

- 4 sourdough bread slices
- 2 tbsp mayonnaise
- 2 slices ham
- 2 lettuce leaves
- 1 tomato, sliced

- 2 mozzarella cheese slices
- Salt and black pepper to taste

Directions:

1. On a clean board, lay the sourdough slices and spread with mayonnaise. Top 2 of the slices with ham, lettuce, tomato and mozzarella. Season with salt and pepper. Top with the remaining two slices to form two sandwiches. Spray with oil and transfer to the frying basket. Cook in the preheated oven for 14 minutes at 340 F on Bake function.

61. Choco Chip Banana Bread

Servings: 10

Cooking Time: 50 Minutes

Ingredients:

- 2 eggs
- 3 ripe bananas
- 1 tsp vanilla
- 1 cup granulated sugar
- 1/2 cup sour cream
- 1/2 cup butter, melted
- 1/2 cup chocolate chips
- 1 1/2 cups all-purpose flour
- 1 tsp baking soda
- 1 tsp salt

Directions:

1. Fit the oven with the rack in position
2. In a large bowl, add bananas and mash using a fork until smooth.
3. Stir in sour cream and melted butter.
4. Add eggs, vanilla, sugar, and salt and stir well.
5. Add flour, baking soda, and salt and stir until just combined.
6. Add chocolate chips and stir well.
7. Pour batter into the greased 9*8-inch loaf pan.
8. Set to bake at 350 F for 55 minutes, after 5 minutes, place the loaf pan in the oven.
9. Slice and serve.

- **Nutrition Info:** Calories 339 Fat 15.3 g Carbohydrates 48 g Sugar 28.9 g Protein 4.5 g Cholesterol 64 mg

62. Creamy Potato Gratin With Nutmeg

Servings:4

Cooking Time: 30 Minutes

Ingredients:

- 1 lb potatoes, peeled and sliced
- ½ cup sour cream
- ½ cup mozzarella cheese, grated
- ½ cup milk
- ½ tsp nutmeg
- Salt and black pepper to taste

Directions:

1. Preheat on Bake function to 390 F. In a bowl, combine sour cream, milk, pepper, salt, and nutmeg. Place the potato slices in the bowl with the milk mixture and stir to coat well.
2. Transfer the mixture to a baking dish and press Start. Cook for 20 minutes, then sprinkle grated cheese on top and cook for 5 more minutes. Serve warm.

63. Almond & Cinnamon Berry Oat Bars

Servings: 10

Cooking Time: 40 Minutes

Ingredients:

- 3 cups rolled oats
- ½ cup ground almonds
- ½ cup flour
- 1 tsp baking powder
- 1 tsp ground cinnamon
- 3 eggs, lightly beaten
- ½ cup canola oil
- ⅓ cup milk
- 2 tsp vanilla extract
- 2 cups mixed berries

Directions:

1. Spray the baking pan with cooking spray. In a bowl, add oats, almonds, flour, baking powder and cinnamon into and stir well. In another bowl, whisk eggs, oil, milk, and vanilla.
2. Stir the wet ingredients gently into the oat mixture. Fold in the berries. Pour the mixture in the pan and place in the toaster oven. Cook for 15-20 minutes at 350 F on Bake function until is nice and soft. Let cool and cut into bars to serve.

64. Brioche Breakfast Pudding

Servings: 8

Cooking Time: 45 Minutes

Ingredients:

- 1 loaf brioche bread, cut in cubes
- ½ tbsp. coconut oil, soft
- 4 cups milk
- 1 can coconut milk
- 6 eggs
- ½ cup sugar
- 2 tsp vanilla
- ¼ tsp salt
- 1 cup coconut, shredded
- ½ cup chocolate chips

Directions:

1. Place rack in position 1 of the oven. Grease an 8x11-inch baking pan with coconut oil.
2. Add the bread cubes to the pan, pressing lightly to settle.
3. In a large bowl, whisk together milk, coconut milk, eggs, sugar, vanilla, and salt until combined.
4. Stir in coconut and chocolate chips. Pour evenly over bread. Cover with plastic wrap and refrigerate 2 hours or overnight.
5. Set oven to bake on 350°F for 50 minutes. After 5 minutes, add the pudding to the oven and bake 40-45 minutes, or until top is beginning to brown and it passes the toothpick test.
6. Remove to wire rack and let cool 5-10 minutes before serving.

- **Nutrition Info:** Calories 476, Total Fat 24g, Saturated Fat 15g, Total Carbs 51g, Net Carbs 48g, Protein 14g, Sugar 30g, Fiber 3g, Sodium 398mg, Potassium 443mg, Phosphorus 288mg

65. Middle Eastern Shakshuka With Smoked Paprika

Servings:x

Cooking Time:x

Ingredients:

- 2 Tbsp olive oil
- ½ yellow onion, diced
- 1 small serrano or jalapeno chili, seeds removed, diced
- 1 tsp cumin
- 1 tsp paprika
- ½ tsp smoked paprika
- ¼ tsp coriander
- 2 eggs
- 1 can chopped tomatoes
- ½ green pepper, diced
- Salt and pepper, to taste
- Chopped parsley or cilantro

Directions:

1. Preheat oven over medium heat.
2. Heat olive oil and saute onion until softened.
3. Add tomatoes, green pepper and chili. Cook for 4-5 minutes.
4. Add seasonings and cook for several minutes until liquid slightly reduces.
5. Make two indentations in mixture and crack eggs into them. Cover and
6. cook until eggs are done.
7. Sprinkle with salt, pepper, parsley and cilantro and serve while bubbly and hot.

66. Egg & Bacon Wraps With Salsa

Servings:3

Cooking Time: 15 Minutes

Ingredients:

- 3 tortillas
- 2 previously scrambled eggs
- 3 slices bacon, cut into strips
- 3 tbsp salsa
- 3 tbsp cream cheese
- 1 cup Pepper Jack cheese, grated

Directions:

1. Preheat on AirFry function to 390 F. Spread 1 tbsp of cream cheese onto each tortilla. Divide the eggs and bacon between the tortillas evenly. Top with salsa and sprinkle some grated cheese over. Roll up the tortillas and press Start. Cook for 10 minutes. Serve.

67. Breakfast Sandwich

Servings: 1

Cooking Time: 7minutes

Ingredients:

- 2 Bacon Slices
- 1 Egg
- 1 English muffin Salt& Pepper to taste

Directions:

1. Beat the egg into a soufflé cup and add salt and pepper to taste.

2. Heat the air fryer to 390°F and place the soufflé cup, English muffin and bacon into the tray.
3. Cook all the ingredients for 6-10 minutes. Assemble sandwich and enjoy.

- **Nutrition Info:** Calories 113 Fat 8.2 g Carbohydrates 0.3 g Sugar 0.2 g Protein 5.4 g Cholesterol 18 mg

68. Cinnamon & Vanilla Toast

Servings:6
Cooking Time: 10 Minutes
Ingredients:

- 12 bread slices
- ½ cup sugar
- 1 ½ tsp cinnamon
- 1 stick of butter, softened
- 1 tsp vanilla extract

Directions:

1. Preheat on Toast function to 300 F. Combine all ingredients, except the bread, in a bowl. Spread the buttery cinnamon mixture onto the bread slices. Place the bread slices in the oven and press Start. Cook for 8 minutes. Serve.

69. Spinach Zucchini Egg Muffins

Servings: 12
Cooking Time: 20 Minutes
Ingredients:

- 8 eggs
- 1 cup baby spinach, chopped
- 1 red bell pepper, diced
- 1/4 cup green onion, chopped
- 12 bacon slices, cooked and crumbled
- 2 small zucchini, sliced
- 1/4 cup almond milk
- 2 tbsp parsley, chopped
- 1 tbsp olive oil
- Pepper
- Salt

Directions:

1. Fit the oven with the rack in position
2. Spray 12-cups muffin tin with cooking spray and set aside.
3. Heat olive oil in a pan over medium heat.
4. Add parsley, spinach, green onion, red bell pepper to the pan and sauté until spinach is wilted.
5. In a bowl, whisk eggs with almond milk, pepper, and salt.
6. Add sautéed vegetables, bacon, and zucchini to the egg mixture and stir well.
7. Pour egg mixture into the greased muffin tin.
8. Set to bake at 350 F for 25 minutes, after 5 minutes, place muffin tin in the oven.
9. Serve and enjoy.

- **Nutrition Info:** Calories 174 Fat 13.3 g Carbohydrates 2.5 g Sugar 1.3 g Protein 11.3 g Cholesterol 130 mg

70. Easy Cheesy Breakfast Casserole

Servings: 8
Cooking Time: 30 Minutes
Ingredients:

- 6 eggs, lightly beaten
- 8 oz can crescent rolls
- 2 cups cheddar cheese, shredded
- 1 lb breakfast sausage, cooked

Directions:

1. Fit the oven with the rack in position
2. Spray a 9*13-inch baking dish with cooking spray and set aside.
3. Spread crescent rolls in the bottom of the prepared baking dish and top with sausage, egg, and cheese.
4. Set to bake at 350 F for 35 minutes. After 5 minutes place the baking dish in the preheated oven.
5. Serve and enjoy.

- **Nutrition Info:** Calories 465 Fat 34.6 g Carbohydrates 11.8 g Sugar 2.4 g Protein 24.2 g Cholesterol 200 mg

71. Blueberry Cake

Servings:8
Cooking Time: 10 Minutes
Ingredients:

- 1½ cups Bisquick
- ¼ cup granulated sugar
- 2 large eggs, beaten
- ¾ cup whole milk
- 1 teaspoon vanilla extract

- ½ teaspoon lemon zest
- Cooking spray
- 2 cups blueberries

Directions:

1. Stir together the Bisquick and sugar in a medium bowl. Stir together the eggs, milk, vanilla and lemon zest. Add the wet ingredients to the dry ingredients and stir until well combined.
2. Spritz the baking pan with cooking spray and line with parchment paper, pressing it into place. Spray the parchment paper with cooking spray. Pour the batter into the pan and spread it out evenly. Sprinkle the blueberries evenly over the top.
3. Slide the baking pan into Rack Position 1, select Convection Bake, set temperature to 375ºF (190ºC) and set time to 10 minutes.
4. When cooking is complete, the cake should be pulling away from the edges of the pan and the top should be just starting to turn golden brown.
5. Let the cake rest for a minute before cutting into 16 squares. Serve immediately.

72. Zucchini And Carrot Pudding

Servings: 4

Cooking Time: 15 Minutes

Ingredients:

- 1 cup carrots, shredded
- 1 cup zucchinis, grated
- 1 cup heavy cream
- 1 cup wild rice
- 2 cups coconut milk
- 1 teaspoon cardamom, ground
- 2 teaspoons sugar
- Cooking spray

Directions:

1. Spray your air fryer with cooking spray, add the carrots, zucchinis and the other ingredients, toss, cover and cook at 365 degrees F for 15 minutes.
2. Divide the pudding into bowls and serve for breakfast.

- **Nutrition Info:** calories 172, fat 7, fiber 4, carbs 14, protein 5

73. Crunchy Asparagus With Cheese

Servings: 4

Cooking Time: 15 Minutes

Ingredients:

- 1 lb asparagus spears
- ¼ cup flour
- 1 cup breadcrumbs
- ½ cup Parmesan cheese, grated
- 2 eggs, beaten
- Salt and black pepper to taste

Directions:

1. Preheat on Air Fry function to 370 F. Combine the breadcrumbs and Parmesan cheese in a bowl. Season with salt and pepper.
2. Line a baking sheet with parchment paper. Dip the asparagus spears into the flour first, then into the eggs, and finally coat with crumbs.
3. Arrange them on the AirFryer Basket, fit in the baking sheet, and cook for about 8 to 10 minutes. Serve with melted butter, hollandaise sauce, or freshly squeezed lemon.

74. Salsa Verde Golden Chicken Empanadas

Servings: 12 Empanadas

Cooking Time: 12 Minutes

Ingredients:

- 1 cup boneless, skinless rotisserie chicken breast meat, chopped finely
- ¼ cup salsa verde
- $^{2}/_{3}$ cup shredded Cheddar cheese
- 1 teaspoon ground cumin
- 1 teaspoon ground black pepper
- 2 purchased refrigerated pie crusts, from a minimum 14.1-ounce (400 g) box
- 1 large egg
- 2 tablespoons water
- Cooking spray

Directions:

1. Spritz the air fryer basket with cooking spray. Set aside.
2. Combine the chicken meat, salsa verde, Cheddar, cumin, and black pepper in a large bowl. Stir to mix well. Set aside.

3. Unfold the pie crusts on a clean work surface, then use a large cookie cutter to cut out 3½-inch circles as much as possible.
4. Roll the remaining crusts to a ball and flatten into a circle which has the same thickness of the original crust. Cut out more 3½-inch circles until you have 12 circles in total.
5. Make the empanadas: Divide the chicken mixture in the middle of each circle, about 1½ tablespoons each. Dab the edges of the circle with water. Fold the circle in half over the filling to shape like a half-moon and press to seal, or you can press with a fork.
6. Whisk the egg with water in a small bowl.
7. Arrange the empanadas in the pan and spritz with cooking spray. Brush with whisked egg.
8. Put the air fryer basket on the baking pan and slide into Rack Position 2, select Air Fry, set temperature to 350ºF (180ºC) and set time to 12 minutes.
9. Flip the empanadas halfway through the cooking time.
10. When cooking is complete, the empanadas will be golden and crispy.
11. Serve immediately.

75. Easy Zucchini Frittata

Servings: 4
Cooking Time: 30 Minutes
Ingredients:

- 8 eggs
- 2 zucchinis, chopped and cooked
- 1 tbsp fresh parsley, chopped
- 3 tbsp cheddar cheese, grated
- 1/2 tsp Italian seasoning
- Pepper
- Salt

Directions:

1. Fit the oven with the rack in position
2. In a bowl, whisk eggs with Italian seasoning, pepper, and salt.
3. Add parsley, cheese, and zucchini and stir well.
4. Pour egg mixture into the greased baking dish.
5. Set to bake at 350 F for 35 minutes. After 5 minutes place the baking dish in the preheated oven.
6. Serve and enjoy.

- **Nutrition Info:** Calories 165 Fat 10.9 g Carbohydrates 4.2 g Sugar 2.5 g Protein 13.6 g Cholesterol 333 mg

76. Basil Dill Egg Muffins

Servings: 6
Cooking Time: 20 Minutes
Ingredients:

- 6 eggs
- 1 tbsp chives, chopped
- 1 tbsp fresh basil, chopped
- 1 tbsp fresh cilantro, chopped
- 1/4 cup mozzarella cheese, grated
- 1 tbsp fresh dill, chopped
- 1 tbsp fresh parsley, chopped
- Pepper
- Salt

Directions:

1. Fit the oven with the rack in position
2. Spray 6-cups muffin tin with cooking spray and set aside.
3. In a bowl, whisk eggs with pepper and salt.
4. Add remaining ingredients and stir well.
5. Pour egg mixture into the prepared muffin tin.
6. Set to bake at 350 F for 25 minutes. After 5 minutes place muffin tin in the preheated oven.
7. Serve and enjoy.

- **Nutrition Info:** Calories 68 Fat 4.6 g Carbohydrates 0.8 g Sugar 0.4 g Protein 6 g Cholesterol 164 mg

77. Tasty Cheddar Omelet

Servings: 1
Cooking Time: 20 Minutes
Ingredients:

- 2 eggs
- 2 tbsp cheddar cheese, grated
- 1 tsp soy sauce
- ½ onion, sliced
- Salt and black pepper to taste
- 1 tbsp olive oil

Directions:

1. Preheat on Bake function to 350 F. Whisk the eggs with soy sauce, salt, and pepper. Stir in onion. Grease a baking dish with the olive oil and add in the egg mixture. Cook for 10-14 minutes. Top with the grated cheddar cheese and serve.

78. Nutmeg Potato Gratin

Servings: 5

Cooking Time: 45 Minutes

Ingredients:

- 5 large potatoes
- ½ cup sour cream
- ½ cup grated cheese
- ½ cup milk
- ½ tsp nutmeg
- Salt and black pepper to taste

Directions:

1. Preheat on Bake function to 375 F, peel and slice the potatoes. In a bowl, combine the sour cream, milk, pepper, salt, and nutmeg. Add in the potato slices and stir to coat them well.
2. Transfer the mixture to an ovenproof casserole. Cook for 15 minutes on Bake function, then sprinkle the cheese on top and cook for 10 minutes. Allow to sit for 10 minutes before serving.

LUNCH RECIPES

79. Boneless Air Fryer Turkey Breasts

Servings: 4
Cooking Time: 50 Minutes
Ingredients:

- 3 lb boneless breast
- ¼ cup mayonnaise
- 2 tsp poultry seasoning
- 1 tsp salt
- ½ tsp garlic powder
- ¼ tsp black pepper

Directions:

1. Choose the Air Fry option on the Instant Pot Duo Crisp Air fryer. Set the temperature to 360°F and push start. The preheating will start.
2. Season your boneless turkey breast with mayonnaise, poultry seasoning, salt, garlic powder, and black pepper.
3. Once preheated, Air Fry the turkey breasts on 360°F for 1 hour, turning every 15 minutes or until internal temperature has reached a temperature of 165°F.

- **Nutrition Info:** Calories 558, Total Fat 18g, Total Carbs 1g, Protein 98g

80. Bok Choy And Butter Sauce(1)

Servings: 4
Cooking Time: 12 Minutes
Ingredients:

- 2 bok choy heads; trimmed and cut into strips
- 1 tbsp. butter; melted
- 2 tbsp. chicken stock
- 1 tsp. lemon juice
- 1 tbsp. olive oil
- A pinch of salt and black pepper

Directions:

1. In a pan that fits your air fryer, mix all the ingredients, toss, introduce the pan in the air fryer and cook at 380°F for 15 minutes.
2. Divide between plates and serve as a side dish

- **Nutrition Info:** Calories: 141; Fat: 3g; Fiber: 2g; Carbs: 4g; Protein: 3g

81. Sweet Potato And Eggplant Mix

Servings: 4
Cooking Time: 20 Minutes
Ingredients:

- 2 sweet potatoes, peeled and cut into medium wedges
- 2 eggplants, roughly cubed
- 1 tablespoon avocado oil
- Juice of 1 lemon
- 4 garlic cloves, minced
- 1 teaspoon nutmeg, ground
- Salt and black pepper to the taste
- 1 tablespoon rosemary, chopped

Directions:

1. In your air fryer, combine the potatoes with the eggplants and the other Ingredients:, toss and cook at 370 degrees F for 20 minutes.
2. Divide the mix between plates and serve as a side dish.

- **Nutrition Info:** Calories 182, fat 6, fiber 3, carbs 11, protein 5

82. Rolled Salmon Sandwich

Servings: 1
Cooking Time: 5 Minutes
Ingredients:

- 1 piece of flatbread
- 1 salmon filet
- Pinch of salt
- 1 tablespoon green onion, chopped
- 1/4 teaspoon dried sumac
- 1/2 teaspoon thyme
- 1/2 teaspoon sesame seeds
- 1/4 English cucumber
- 1 tablespoon yogurt

Directions:

1. Start by peeling and chopping the cucumber. Cut the salmon at a 45-degree angle into 4 slices and lay them flat on the flatbread.
2. Sprinkle salmon with salt to taste. Sprinkle onions, thyme, sumac, and sesame seeds evenly over the salmon.
3. Broil the salmon for at least 3 minutes, but longer if you want a more well-done fish.

4. While you broil your salmon, mix together the yogurt and cucumber. Remove your flatbread from the toaster oven and put it on a plate, then spoon the yogurt mix over the salmon.
5. Fold the sides of the flatbread in and roll it up for a gourmet lunch that you can take on the go.

- **Nutrition Info:** Calories: 347, Sodium: 397 mg, Dietary Fiber: 1.6 g, Total Fat: 12.4 g, Total Carbs: 20.6 g, Protein: 38.9 g.

83. Spicy Green Crusted Chicken

Servings: 6
Cooking Time: 40 Minutes

Ingredients:

- 6 eggs, beaten
- 6 teaspoons parsley
- 4 teaspoons thyme
- 1 pound chicken pieces
- 6 teaspoons oregano
- Salt and freshly ground black pepper, to taste
- 4 teaspoons paprika

Directions:

1. Preheat the Air fryer to 360 degree F and grease an Air fryer basket.
2. Whisk eggs in a bowl and mix all the ingredients in another bowl except chicken pieces.
3. Dip the chicken in eggs and then coat generously with the dry mixture.
4. Arrange half of the chicken pieces in the Air fryer basket and cook for about 20 minutes.
5. Repeat with the remaining mixture and dish out to serve hot.

- **Nutrition Info:** Calories: 218, Fat: 10.4g, Carbohydrates: 2.6g, Sugar: 0.6g, Protein: 27.9g, Sodium: 128mg

84. Chicken & Rice Casserole

Servings: 6
Cooking Time: 40 Minutes

Ingredients:

- 2 lbs. bone-in chicken thighs
- Salt and black pepper
- 1 teaspoon olive oil
- 5 cloves garlic, chopped
- 2 large onions, chopped
- 2 large red bell peppers, chopped
- 1 tablespoon sweet Hungarian paprika
- 1 teaspoon hot Hungarian paprika
- 2 tablespoons tomato paste
- 2 cups chicken broth
- 3 cups brown rice, thawed
- 2 tablespoons parsley, chopped
- 6 tablespoons sour cream

Directions:

1. Mix broth, tomato paste, and all the spices in a bowl.
2. Add chicken and mix well to coat.
3. Spread the rice in a casserole dish and add chicken along with its marinade.
4. Top the casserole with the rest of the Ingredients:.
5. Press "Power Button" of Air Fry Oven and turn the dial to select the "Bake" mode.
6. Press the Time button and again turn the dial to set the cooking time to 40 minutes.
7. Now push the Temp button and rotate the dial to set the temperature at 350 degrees F.
8. Once preheated, place the baking pan inside and close its lid.
9. Serve warm.

- **Nutrition Info:** Calories 440 Total Fat 7.9 g Saturated Fat 1.8 g Cholesterol 5 mg Sodium 581 mg Total Carbs 21.8 g Sugar 7.1 g Fiber 2.6 g Protein 37.2 g

85. Roasted Mini Peppers

Servings: 6
Cooking Time: 15 Minutes

Ingredients:

- 1 bag mini bell peppers
- Cooking spray
- Salt and pepper to taste

Directions:

1. Start by preheating toaster oven to 400°F.
2. Wash and dry the peppers, then place flat on a baking sheet.
3. Spray peppers with cooking spray and sprinkle with salt and pepper.
4. Roast for 15 minutes.

- **Nutrition Info:** Calories: 19, Sodium: 2 mg, Dietary Fiber: 1.3 g, Total Fat: 0.3 g, Total Carbs: 3.6 g, Protein: 0.6 g.

86. Chives Radishes

Servings: 4
Cooking Time: 12 Minutes
Ingredients:

- 20 radishes; halved
- 2 tbsp. olive oil
- 1 tbsp. garlic; minced
- 1 tsp. chives; chopped.
- Salt and black pepper to taste.

Directions:

1. In your air fryer's pan, combine all the ingredients and toss.
2. Introduce the pan in the machine and cook at 370°F for 15 minutes
3. Divide between plates and serve as a side dish.

- **Nutrition Info:** Calories: 160; Fat: 2g; Fiber: 3g; Carbs: 4g; Protein: 6g

87. Amazing Mac And Cheese

Servings:
Cooking Time: 12 Minutes
Ingredients:

- 1 cup cooked macaroni
- 1/2 cup warm milk
- 1 tablespoon parmesan cheese
- 1 cup grated cheddar cheese
- salt and pepper; to taste

Directions:

1. Preheat the Air Fryer to 350 - degrees Fahrenheit. Stir all of the ingredients; except Parmesan, in a baking dish.
2. Place the dish inside the Air Fryer and cook for 10 minutes. Top with the Parmesan cheese.

88. Kalamta Mozarella Pita Melts

Servings: 2
Cooking Time: 5 Minutes
Ingredients:

- 2 (6-inch) whole wheat pitas
- 1 teaspoon extra-virgin olive oil
- 1 cup grated part-skim mozzarella cheese
- 1/4 small red onion
- 1/4 cup pitted Kalamata olives
- 2 tablespoons chopped fresh herbs such as parsley, basil, or oregano

Directions:

1. Start by preheating toaster oven to 425°F.
2. Brush the pita on both sides with oil and warm in the oven for one minute.
3. Dice onions and halve olives.
4. Sprinkle mozzarella over each pita and top with onion and olive.
5. Return to the oven for another 5 minutes or until the cheese is melted.
6. Sprinkle herbs over the pita and serve.

- **Nutrition Info:** Calories: 387, Sodium: 828 mg, Dietary Fiber: 7.4 g, Total Fat: 16.2 g, Total Carbs: 42.0 g, Protein: 23.0 g.

89. Chicken Wings With Prawn Paste

Servings: 6
Cooking Time: 8 Minutes
Ingredients:

- Corn flour, as required
- 2 pounds mid-joint chicken wings
- 2 tablespoons prawn paste
- 4 tablespoons olive oil
- 1½ teaspoons sugar
- 2 teaspoons sesame oil
- 1 teaspoon Shaoxing wine
- 2 teaspoons fresh ginger juice

Directions:

1. Preheat the Air fryer to 360 degree F and grease an Air fryer basket.
2. Mix all the ingredients in a bowl except wings and corn flour.
3. Rub the chicken wings generously with marinade and refrigerate overnight.
4. Coat the chicken wings evenly with corn flour and keep aside.
5. Set the Air fryer to 390 degree F and arrange the chicken wings in the Air fryer basket.
6. Cook for about 8 minutes and dish out to serve hot.

- **Nutrition Info:** Calories: 416, Fat: 31.5g, Carbohydrates: 11.2g, Sugar: 1.6g, Protein: 24.4g, Sodium: 661mg

90. Pumpkin Pancakes

Servings: 4
Cooking Time: 12 Minutes
Ingredients:

- 1 square puff pastry
- 3 tablespoons pumpkin filling
- 1 small egg, beaten

Directions:

1. Roll out a square of puff pastry and layer it with pumpkin pie filling, leaving about ¼-inch space around the edges.
2. Cut it up into 8 equal sized square pieces and coat the edges with beaten egg.
3. Press "Power Button" of Air Fry Oven and turn the dial to select the "Air Fry" mode.
4. Press the Time button and again turn the dial to set the cooking time to 12 minutes.
5. Now push the Temp button and rotate the dial to set the temperature at 355 degrees F.
6. Press "Start/Pause" button to start.
7. When the unit beeps to show that it is preheated, open the lid.
8. Arrange the squares into a greased "Sheet Pan" and insert in the oven.
9. Serve warm.

- **Nutrition Info:** Calories: 109 Cal Total Fat: 6.7 g Saturated Fat: 1.8 g Cholesterol: 34 mg Sodium: 87 mg Total Carbs: 9.8 g Fiber: 0.5 g Sugar: 2.6 g Protein: 2.4 g

91. Chicken With Veggies And Rice

Servings: 3
Cooking Time: 20 Minutes
Ingredients:

- 3 cups cold boiled white rice
- 1 cup cooked chicken, diced
- ½ cup frozen carrots
- ½ cup frozen peas
- ½ cup onion, chopped
- 6 tablespoons soy sauce
- 1 tablespoon vegetable oil

Directions:

1. Preheat the Air fryer to 360 degree F and grease a 7" nonstick pan.
2. Mix the rice, soy sauce, and vegetable oil in a bowl.
3. Stir in the remaining ingredients and mix until well combined.
4. Transfer the rice mixture into the pan and place in the Air fryer.
5. Cook for about 20 minutes and dish out to serve immediately.

- **Nutrition Info:** Calories: 405, Fat: 6.4g, Carbohydrates: 63g, Sugar: 3.5g, Protein: 21.7g, Sodium: 1500mg

92. Simple Turkey Breast

Servings: 10
Cooking Time: 40 Minutes
Ingredients:

- 1: 8-poundsbone-in turkey breast
- Salt and black pepper, as required
- 2 tablespoons olive oil

Directions:

1. Preheat the Air fryer to 360 degree F and grease an Air fryer basket.
2. Season the turkey breast with salt and black pepper and drizzle with oil.
3. Arrange the turkey breast into the Air Fryer basket, skin side down and cook for about 20 minutes.
4. Flip the side and cook for another 20 minutes.
5. Dish out in a platter and cut into desired size slices to serve.

- **Nutrition Info:** Calories: 719, Fat: 35.9g, Carbohydrates: 0g, Sugar: 0g, Protein: 97.2g, Sodium: 386mg

93. Deviled Chicken

Servings: 8
Cooking Time: 40 Minutes
Ingredients:

- 2 tablespoons butter
- 2 cloves garlic, chopped
- 1 cup Dijon mustard
- 1/2 teaspoon cayenne pepper
- 1 1/2 cups panko breadcrumbs
- 3/4 cup Parmesan, freshly grated
- 1/4 cup chives, chopped
- 2 teaspoons paprika
- 8 small bone-in chicken thighs, skin removed

Directions:

1. Toss the chicken thighs with crumbs, cheese, chives, butter, and spices in a bowl and mix well to coat.
2. Transfer the chicken along with its spice mix to a baking pan.

3. Press "Power Button" of Air Fry Oven and turn the dial to select the "Air Fry" mode.
4. Press the Time button and again turn the dial to set the cooking time to 40 minutes.
5. Now push the Temp button and rotate the dial to set the temperature at 350 degrees F.
6. Once preheated, place the baking pan inside and close its lid.
7. Serve warm.

- **Nutrition Info:** Calories 380 Total Fat 20 g Saturated Fat 5 g Cholesterol 151 mg Sodium 686 mg Total Carbs 33 g Fiber 1 g Sugar 1.2 g Protein 21 g

94. Philly Cheesesteak Egg Rolls

Servings: 4-5
Cooking Time: 20 Minutes
Ingredients:

- 1 egg
- 1 tablespoon milk
- 2 tablespoons olive oil
- 1 small red onion
- 1 small red bell pepper
- 1 small green bell pepper
- 1 pound thinly slice roast beef
- 8 ounces shredded pepper jack cheese
- 8 ounces shredded provolone cheese
- 8-10 egg roll skins
- Salt and pepper

Directions:

1. Start by preheating toaster oven to 425°F.
2. Mix together egg and milk in a shallow bowl and set aside for later use.
3. Chop onions and bell peppers into small pieces.
4. Heat the oil in a medium sauce pan and add the onions and peppers.
5. Cook onions and peppers for 2–3 minutes until softened.
6. Add roast beef to the pan and sauté for another 5 minutes.
7. Add salt and pepper to taste.
8. Add cheese and mix together until melted.
9. Remove from heat and drain liquid from pan.
10. Roll the egg roll skins flat.
11. Add equal parts of the mix to each egg roll and roll them up per the instructions on the package.
12. Brush each egg roll with the egg mixture.
13. Line a pan with parchment paper and lay egg rolls seam-side down with a gap between each roll.
14. Bake for 20–25 minutes, depending on your preference of egg roll crispness.

- **Nutrition Info:** Calories: 769, Sodium: 1114 mg, Dietary Fiber: 2.1 g, Total Fat: 39.9 g, Total Carbs: 41.4 g, Protein: 58.4 g.

95. Jicama Fries(1)

Servings: 4
Cooking Time: 12 Minutes
Ingredients:

- 1 small jicama; peeled.
- ¼ tsp. onion powder.
- ¾tsp. chili powder
- ¼ tsp. ground black pepper
- ¼ tsp. garlic powder.

Directions:

1. Cut jicama into matchstick-sized pieces.
2. Place pieces into a small bowl and sprinkle with remaining ingredients. Place the fries into the air fryer basket
3. Adjust the temperature to 350 Degrees F and set the timer for 20 minutes. Toss the basket two or three times during cooking. Serve warm.

- **Nutrition Info:** Calories: 37; Protein: 8g; Fiber: 7g; Fat: 1g; Carbs: 7g

96. Pecan Crunch Catfish And Asparagus

Servings: 4
Cooking Time: 12 Minutes
Ingredients:

- 1 cup whole wheat panko breadcrumbs
- 1/4 cup chopped pecans
- 3 teaspoons chopped fresh thyme
- 1-1/2 tablespoons extra-virgin olive oil, plus more for the pan
- Salt and pepper to taste
- 1-1/4 pounds asparagus
- 1 tablespoon honey
- 4 (5- to 6-ounce each) catfish filets

Directions:

1. Start by preheating toaster oven to 425°F.
2. Combine breadcrumbs, pecans, 2 teaspoons thyme, 1 tablespoon oil, salt, pepper and 2 tablespoons water.
3. In another bowl combine asparagus, the rest of the thyme, honey, salt, and pepper.
4. Spread the asparagus in a flat layer on a baking sheet. Sprinkle a quarter of the breadcrumb mixture over the asparagus.
5. Lay the catfish over the asparagus and press the rest of the breadcrumb mixture into each piece. Roast for 12 minutes.

- **Nutrition Info:** Calories: 531, Sodium: 291 mg, Dietary Fiber: 6.1 g, Total Fat: 30.4 g, Total Carbs: 31.9 g, Protein: 34.8 g.

97. Pork Stew

Servings: 4
Cooking Time: 12 Minutes
Ingredients:

- 2 lb. pork stew meat; cubed
- 1 eggplant; cubed
- ½ cup beef stock
- 2 zucchinis; cubed
- ½ tsp. smoked paprika
- Salt and black pepper to taste.
- A handful cilantro; chopped.

Directions:

1. In a pan that fits your air fryer, mix all the ingredients, toss, introduce in your air fryer and cook at 370°F for 30 minutes
2. Divide into bowls and serve right away.

- **Nutrition Info:** Calories: 245; Fat: 12g; Fiber: 2g; Carbs: 5g; Protein: 14g

98. Onion Omelet

Servings: 2
Cooking Time: 15 Minutes
Ingredients:

- 4 eggs
- ¼ teaspoon low-sodium soy sauce
- Ground black pepper, as required
- 1 teaspoon butter
- 1 medium yellow onion, sliced
- ¼ cup Cheddar cheese, grated

Directions:

1. In a skillet, melt the butter over medium heat and cook the onion and cook for about 8-10 minutes.
2. Remove from the heat and set aside to cool slightly.
3. Meanwhile, in a bowl, add the eggs, soy sauce and black pepper and beat well.
4. Add the cooked onion and gently, stir to combine.
5. Place the zucchini mixture into a small baking pan.
6. Press "Power Button" of Air Fry Oven and turn the dial to select the "Air Fry" mode.
7. Press the Time button and again turn the dial to set the cooking time to 5 minutes.
8. Now push the Temp button and rotate the dial to set the temperature at 355 degrees F.
9. Press "Start/Pause" button to start.
10. When the unit beeps to show that it is preheated, open the lid.
11. Arrange pan over the "Wire Rack" and insert in the oven.
12. Cut the omelet into 2 portions and serve hot.

- **Nutrition Info:** Calories: 222 Cal Total Fat: 15.4 g Saturated Fat: 6.9 g Cholesterol: 347 mg Sodium: 264 mg Total Carbs: 6.1 g Fiber: 1.2 g Sugar: 3.1 g Protein: 15.3 g

99. Roasted Stuffed Peppers

Servings: 4
Cooking Time: 20 Minutes
Ingredients:

- 4 ounces shredded cheddar cheese
- ½ tsp. Pepper
- ½ tsp. Salt
- 1 tsp. Worcestershire sauce
- ½ c. Tomato sauce
- 8 ounces lean ground beef
- 1 tsp. Olive oil
- 1 minced garlic clove
- ½ chopped onion
- 2 green peppers

Directions:

1. Preparing the ingredients. Ensure your instant crisp air fryer is preheated to 390 degrees. Spray with olive oil.

2. Cut stems off bell peppers and remove seeds. Cook in boiling salted water for 3 minutes.
3. Sauté garlic and onion together in a skillet until golden in color.
4. Take skillet off the heat. Mix pepper, salt, Worcestershire sauce, ¼ cup of tomato sauce, half of cheese and beef together.
5. Divide meat mixture into pepper halves. Top filled peppers with remaining cheese and tomato sauce.
6. Place filled peppers in the instant crisp air fryer.
7. Air frying. Close air fryer lid. Set temperature to 390°f, and set time to 20 minutes, bake 15-20 minutes.

- **Nutrition Info:** Calories: 295; Fat: 8g; Protein:23g; Sugar:2g

100.Chicken Legs With Dilled Brussels Sprouts

Servings: 2
Cooking Time: 10 Minutes
Ingredients:

- 2 chicken legs
- 1/2 teaspoon paprika
- 1/2 teaspoon kosher salt
- 1/2 teaspoon black pepper
- 1/2 pound Brussels sprouts
- 1 teaspoon dill, fresh or dried

Directions:

1. Start by preheating your Air Fryer to 370 degrees F.
2. Now, season your chicken with paprika, salt, and pepper. Transfer the chicken legs to the cooking basket. Cook for 10 minutes.
3. Flip the chicken legs and cook an additional 10 minutes. Reserve.
4. Add the Brussels sprouts to the cooking basket; sprinkle with dill. Cook at 380 degrees F for 15 minutes, shaking the basket halfway through.
5. Serve with the reserved chicken legs.

- **Nutrition Info:** 365 Calories; 21g Fat; 3g Carbs; 36g Protein; 2g Sugars; 3g Fiber

101.Squash And Zucchini Mini Pizza

Servings: 4
Cooking Time: 15 Minutes
Ingredients:

- 1 pizza crust
- 1/2 cup parmesan cheese
- 4 tablespoons oregano
- 1 zucchini
- 1 yellow summer squash
- Olive oil
- Salt and pepper

Directions:

1. Start by preheating toaster oven to 350°F.
2. If you are using homemade crust, roll out 8 mini portions; if crust is store-bought, use a cookie cutter to cut out the portions.
3. Sprinkle parmesan and oregano equally on each piece. Layer the zucchini and squash in a circle – one on top of the other – around the entire circle.
4. Brush with olive oil and sprinkle salt and pepper to taste.
5. Bake for 15 minutes and serve.

- **Nutrition Info:** Calories: 151, Sodium: 327 mg, Dietary Fiber: 3.1 g, Total Fat: 8.6 g, Total Carbs: 10.3 g, Protein: 11.4 g.

102.Ranch Chicken Wings

Servings: 3
Cooking Time: 10 Minutes
Ingredients:

- 1/4 cup almond meal
- 1/4 cup flaxseed meal
- 2 tablespoons butter, melted
- 6 tablespoons parmesan cheese, preferably freshly grated
- 1 tablespoon Ranch seasoning mix
- 2 tablespoons oyster sauce
- 6 chicken wings, bone-in

Directions:

1. Start by preheating your Air Fryer to 370 degrees F.
2. In a resealable bag, place the almond meal, flaxseed meal, butter, parmesan, Ranch seasoning mix, andoyster sauce. Add the chicken wings and shake to coat on all sides.
3. Arrange the chicken wings in the Air Fryer basket. Spritz the chicken wings with a nonstick cooking spray.

4. Cook for 11 minutes. Turn them over and cook an additional 11 minutes. Serve warm with your favorite dipping sauce, if desired. Enjoy!

- **Nutrition Info:** 285 Calories; 22g Fat; 3g Carbs; 12g Protein; 5g Sugars; 6g Fiber

103.Spicy Egg And Ground Turkey Bake

Servings: 6
Cooking Time: 10 Minutes
Ingredients:

- 1½ pounds ground turkey
- 6 whole eggs, well beaten
- 1/3 teaspoon smoked paprika
- 2 egg whites, beaten
- Tabasco sauce, for drizzling
- 2 tablespoons sesame oil
- 2 leeks, chopped
- 3 cloves garlic, finely minced
- 1 teaspoon ground black pepper
- 1/2 teaspoon sea salt

Directions:

1. Warm the oil in a pan over moderate heat; then, sweat the leeks and garlic until tender; stir periodically.
2. Next, grease 6 oven safe ramekins with pan spray. Divide the sautéed mixture among six ramekins.
3. In a bowl, beat the eggs and egg whites using a wire whisk. Stir in the smoked paprika, salt and black pepper; whisk until everything is thoroughly combined. Divide the egg mixture among the ramekins.
4. Air-fry approximately 22 minutes at 345 degrees F. Drizzle Tabasco sauce over each portion and serve.

- **Nutrition Info:** 298 Calories; 16g Fat; 4g Carbs; 16g Protein; 9g Sugars; 7g Fiber

104.Spicy Avocado Cauliflower Toast

Servings: 2
Cooking Time: 15 Minutes
Ingredients:

- 1/2 large head of cauliflower, leaves removed
- 3 1/4 teaspoons olive oil
- 1 small jalapeño
- 1 tablespoon chopped cilantro leaves
- 2 slices whole grain bread
- 1 medium avocado
- Salt and pepper
- 5 radishes
- 1 green onion
- 2 teaspoons hot sauce
- 1 lime

Directions:

1. Start by preheating toaster oven to 450°F.
2. Cut cauliflower into thick pieces, about 3/4-inches-thick, and slice jalapeño into thin slices.
3. Place cauliflower and jalapeño in a bowl and mix together with 2 teaspoons olive oil.
4. Add salt and pepper to taste and mix for another minute.
5. Coat a pan with another teaspoon of olive oil, then lay the cauliflower mixture flat across the pan.
6. Cook for 20 minutes, flipping in the last 5 minutes.
7. Reduce heat to toast.
8. Sprinkle cilantro over the mix while it is still warm, and set aside.
9. Brush bread with remaining oil and toast until golden brown, about 5 minutes.
10. Dice onion and radish.
11. Mash avocado in a bowl, then spread on toast and sprinkle salt and pepper to taste.
12. Put cauliflower mix on toast and cover with onion and radish. Drizzle with hot sauce and serve with a lime wedge.

- **Nutrition Info:** Calories: 359, Sodium: 308 mg, Dietary Fiber: 11.1 g, Total Fat: 28.3 g, Total Carbs: 26.4 g, Protein: 6.6 g.

105.Turkey And Mushroom Stew

Servings: 4
Cooking Time: 12 Minutes
Ingredients:

- ½ lb. brown mushrooms; sliced
- 1 turkey breast, skinless, boneless; cubed and browned
- ¼ cup tomato sauce
- 1 tbsp. parsley; chopped.
- Salt and black pepper to taste.

Directions:

1. In a pan that fits your air fryer, mix the turkey with the mushrooms, salt, pepper and tomato sauce, toss, introduce in the fryer and cook at 350°F for 25 minutes
2. Divide into bowls and serve for lunch with parsley sprinkled on top.

- **Nutrition Info:** Calories: 220; Fat: 12g; Fiber: 2g; Carbs: 5g; Protein: 12g

106.Lemon Pepper Turkey

Servings: 6

Cooking Time: 45 Minutes

Ingredients:

- 3 lbs. turkey breast
- 2 tablespoons oil
- 1 tablespoon Worcestershire sauce
- 1 teaspoon lemon pepper
- 1/2 teaspoon salt

Directions:

1. Whisk everything in a bowl and coat the turkey liberally.
2. Place the turkey in the Air fryer basket.
3. Press "Power Button" of Air Fry Oven and turn the dial to select the "Air Fry" mode.
4. Press the Time button and again turn the dial to set the cooking time to 45 minutes.
5. Now push the Temp button and rotate the dial to set the temperature at 375 degrees F.
6. Once preheated, place the air fryer basket inside and close its lid.
7. Serve warm.

- **Nutrition Info:** Calories 391 Total Fat 2.8 g Saturated Fat 0.6 g Cholesterol 330 mg Sodium 62 mg Total Carbs 36.5 g Fiber 9.2 g Sugar 4.5 g Protein 6.6

107.Baked Shrimp Scampi

Servings: 4

Cooking Time: 10 Minutes

Ingredients:

- 1 lb large shrimp
- 8 tbsp butter
- 1 tbsp minced garlic (use 2 for extra garlic flavor)
- 1/4 cup white wine or cooking sherry
- 1/2 tsp salt
- 1/4 tsp cayenne pepper
- 1/4 tsp paprika
- 1/2 tsp onion powder
- 3/4 cup bread crumbs

Directions:

1. Take a bowl and mix the bread crumbs with dry seasonings.
2. On the stovetop (or in the Instant Pot on saute), melt the butter with the garlic and the white wine.
3. Remove from heat and add the shrimp and the bread crumb mix.
4. Transfer the mix to a casserole dish.
5. Choose the Bake operation and add food to the Instant Pot Duo Crisp Air Fryer. Close the lid and Bake at 350°F for 10 minutes or until they are browned.
6. Serve and enjoy.

- **Nutrition Info:** Calories 422, Total Fat 26g, Total Carbs 18g, Protein 29 g

108.Turkey Meatloaf

Servings: 4

Cooking Time: 20 Minutes

Ingredients:

- 1 pound ground turkey
- 1 cup kale leaves, trimmed and finely chopped
- 1 cup onion, chopped
- ½ cup fresh breadcrumbs
- 1 cup Monterey Jack cheese, grated
- 2 garlic cloves, minced
- ¼ cup salsa verde
- 1 teaspoon red chili powder
- ½ teaspoon ground cumin
- ½ teaspoon dried oregano, crushed
- Salt and ground black pepper, as required

Directions:

1. Preheat the Air fryer to 400 degree F and grease an Air fryer basket.
2. Mix all the ingredients in a bowl and divide the turkey mixture into 4 equal-sized portions.
3. Shape each into a mini loaf and arrange the loaves into the Air fryer basket.
4. Cook for about 20 minutes and dish out to serve warm.

- **Nutrition Info:** Calories: 435, Fat: 23.1g, Carbohydrates: 18.1g, Sugar: 3.6g, Protein: 42.2g, Sodium: 641mg

109.Eggplant And Leeks Stew

Servings: 4
Cooking Time: 12 Minutes
Ingredients:

- 2 big eggplants, roughly cubed
- ½ bunch cilantro; chopped.
- 1 cup veggie stock
- 2 garlic cloves; minced
- 3 leeks; sliced
- 2 tbsp. olive oil
- 1 tbsp. hot sauce
- 1 tbsp. sweet paprika
- 1 tbsp. tomato puree
- Salt and black pepper to taste.

Directions:

1. In a pan that fits the air fryer, mix all the ingredients, toss, introduce in the fryer and cook at 380°F for 20 minutes
2. Divide the stew into bowls and serve for lunch.

- **Nutrition Info:** Calories: 183; Fat: 4g; Fiber: 2g; Carbs: 4g; Protein: 12g

110.Maple Chicken Thighs

Servings: 4
Cooking Time: 30 Minutes
Ingredients:

- 4 large chicken thighs, bone-in
- 2 tablespoons French mustard
- 2 tablespoons Dijon mustard
- 1 clove minced garlic
- 1/2 teaspoon dried marjoram
- 2 tablespoons maple syrup

Directions:

1. Mix chicken with everything in a bowl and coat it well.
2. Place the chicken along with its marinade in the baking pan.
3. Press "Power Button" of Air Fry Oven and turn the dial to select the "Bake" mode.
4. Press the Time button and again turn the dial to set the cooking time to 30 minutes.
5. Now push the Temp button and rotate the dial to set the temperature at 370 degrees F.
6. Once preheated, place the baking pan inside and close its lid.
7. Serve warm.

- **Nutrition Info:** Calories 301 Total Fat 15.8 g Saturated Fat 2.7 g Cholesterol 75 mg Sodium 189 mg Total Carbs 31.7 g Fiber 0.3 g Sugar 0.1 g Protein 28.2 g

111.Bbq Chicken Breasts

Servings: 4
Cooking Time: 15 Minutes
Ingredients:

- 4 boneless skinless chicken breast about 6 oz each
- 1-2 Tbsp bbq seasoning

Directions:

1. Cover both sides of chicken breast with the BBQ seasoning. Cover and marinate the in the refrigerator for 45 minutes.
2. Choose the Air Fry option and set the temperature to 400°F. Push start and let it preheat for 5 minutes.
3. Upon preheating, place the chicken breast in the Instant Pot Duo Crisp Air Fryer basket, making sure they do not overlap. Spray with oil.
4. Cook for 13-14 minutes
5. flipping halfway.
6. Remove chicken when the chicken reaches an internal temperature of 160°F. Place on a plate and allow to rest for 5 minutes before slicing.

- **Nutrition Info:** Calories 131, Total Fat 3g, Total Carbs 2g, Protein 24g

112.Okra And Green Beans Stew

Servings: 4
Cooking Time: 12 Minutes
Ingredients:

- 1 lb. green beans; halved
- 4 garlic cloves; minced
- 1 cup okra
- 3 tbsp. tomato sauce
- 1 tbsp. thyme; chopped.
- Salt and black pepper to taste.

Directions:

1. In a pan that fits your air fryer, mix all the ingredients, toss, introduce the pan in the air fryer and cook at 370°F for 15 minutes
2. Divide the stew into bowls and serve.

- **Nutrition Info:** Calories: 183; Fat: 5g; Fiber: 2g; Carbs: 4g; Protein: 8g

113.Sweet Potato And Parsnip Spiralized Latkes

Servings: 12
Cooking Time: 20 Minutes
Ingredients:

- 1 medium sweet potato
- 1 large parsnip
- 4 cups water
- 1 egg + 1 egg white
- 2 scallions
- 1/2 teaspoon garlic powder
- 1/2 teaspoon sea salt
- 1/2 teaspoon ground pepper

Directions:

1. Start by spiralizing the sweet potato and parsnip and chopping the scallions, reserving only the green parts.
2. Preheat toaster oven to 425°F.
3. Bring 4 cups of water to a boil. Place all of your noodles in a colander and pour the boiling water over the top, draining well.
4. Let the noodles cool, then grab handfuls and place them in a paper towel; squeeze to remove as much liquid as possible.
5. In a large bowl, beat egg and egg white together. Add noodles, scallions, garlic powder, salt, and pepper, mix well.
6. Prepare a baking sheet; scoop out 1/4 cup of mixture at a time and place on sheet.
7. Slightly press down each scoop with your hands, then bake for 20 minutes, flipping halfway through.

- **Nutrition Info:** Calories: 24, Sodium: 91 mg, Dietary Fiber: 1.0 g, Total Fat: 0.4 g, Total Carbs: 4.3 g, Protein: 0.9 g.

114.Buttermilk Brined Turkey Breast

Servings: 8
Cooking Time: 20 Minutes
Ingredients:

- ¾ cup brine from a can of olives
- 3½ pounds boneless, skinless turkey breast
- 2 fresh thyme sprigs
- 1 fresh rosemary sprig
- ½ cup buttermilk

Directions:

1. Preheat the Air fryer to 350 degree F and grease an Air fryer basket.
2. Mix olive brine and buttermilk in a bowl until well combined.
3. Place the turkey breast, buttermilk mixture and herb sprigs in a resealable plastic bag.
4. Seal the bag and refrigerate for about 12 hours.
5. Remove the turkey breast from bag and arrange the turkey breast into the Air fryer basket.
6. Cook for about 20 minutes, flipping once in between.
7. Dish out the turkey breast onto a cutting board and cut into desired size slices to serve.

- **Nutrition Info:** Calories: 215, Fat: 3.5g, Carbohydrates: 9.4g, Sugar: 7.7g, Protein: 34.4g, Sodium: 2000mg

115.Cheese-stuffed Meatballs

Servings: 4
Cooking Time: 10 Minutes
Ingredients:

- ⅓ cup soft bread crumbs
- 3 tablespoons milk
- 1 tablespoon ketchup
- 1 egg
- ½ teaspoon dried marjoram
- Pinch salt
- Freshly ground black pepper
- 1-pound 95 percent lean ground beef
- 20 ½-inch cubes of cheese
- Olive oil for misting

Directions:

1. Preparing the ingredients. In a large bowl, combine the bread crumbs, milk, ketchup, egg, marjoram, salt, and pepper, and mix well. Add the ground beef and mix gently but thoroughly with your hands. Form the mixture into 20 meatballs. Shape each meatball around a cheese cube. Mist the meatballs with olive oil and put into the instant crisp air fryer basket.
2. Air frying. Close air fryer lid. Bake for 10 to 13 minutes or until the meatballs register 165°f on a meat thermometer.

- **Nutrition Info:** Calories: 393; Fat: 17g; Protein:50g; Fiber:0g

116.Okra Casserole

Servings: 4
Cooking Time: 12 Minutes
Ingredients:

- 2 red bell peppers; cubed
- 2 tomatoes; chopped.
- 3 garlic cloves; minced
- 3 cups okra
- ½ cup cheddar; shredded
- ¼ cup tomato puree
- 1 tbsp. cilantro; chopped.
- 1 tsp. olive oil
- 2 tsp. coriander, ground
- Salt and black pepper to taste.

Directions:

1. Grease a heat proof dish that fits your air fryer with the oil, add all the ingredients except the cilantro and the cheese and toss them really gently
2. Sprinkle the cheese and the cilantro on top, introduce the dish in the fryer and cook at 390°F for 20 minutes.
3. Divide between plates and serve for lunch.

- **Nutrition Info:** Calories: 221; Fat: 7g; Fiber: 2g; Carbs: 4g; Protein: 9g

117.Chicken Potato Bake

Servings: 4
Cooking Time: 25 Minutes
Ingredients:

- 4 potatoes, diced
- 1 tablespoon garlic, minced
- 1.5 tablespoons olive oil
- 1/8 teaspoon salt
- 1/8 teaspoon pepper
- 1.5 lbs. boneless skinless chicken
- 3/4 cup mozzarella cheese, shredded
- parsley chopped

Directions:

1. Toss chicken and potatoes with all the spices and oil in a baking pan.
2. Drizzle the cheese on top of the chicken and potato.
3. Press "Power Button" of Air Fry Oven and turn the dial to select the "Bake" mode.
4. Press the Time button and again turn the dial to set the cooking time to 25 minutes.
5. Now push the Temp button and rotate the dial to set the temperature at 375 degrees F.
6. Once preheated, place the baking pan inside and close its lid.
7. Serve warm.

- **Nutrition Info:** Calories 695 Total Fat 17.5 g Saturated Fat 4.8 g Cholesterol 283 mg Sodium 355 mg Total Carbs 26.4 g Fiber 1.8 g Sugar 0.8 g Protein 117.4 g

DINNER RECIPES

118.Easy Air Fryed Roasted Asparagus

Servings: 4
Cooking Time: 10 Minutes

Ingredients:

- 1 bunch fresh asparagus
- 1 ½ tsp herbs de provence
- Fresh lemon wedge (optional)
- 1 tablespoon olive oil or cooking spray
- Salt and pepper to taste

Directions:

1. Wash asparagus and trim off hard ends
2. Drizzle asparagus with olive oil and add seasonings
3. Place asparagus in air fryer and cook on 360F for 6 to 10 minutes
4. Drizzle squeezed lemon over roasted asparagus.

- **Nutrition Info:** Calories 46 protein 2g fat 3g net carbs 1g

119.Crispy Scallops

Servings: 4
Cooking Time: 6 Minutes

Ingredients:

- 18 sea scallops, cleaned and patted very dry
- 1/8 cup all-purpose flour
- 1 tablespoon 2% milk
- ½ egg
- ¼ cup cornflakes, crushed
- ½ teaspoon paprika
- Salt and black pepper, as required

Directions:

1. Preheat the Air fryer to 400 degree F and grease an Air fryer basket.
2. Mix flour, paprika, salt, and black pepper in a bowl.
3. Whisk egg with milk in another bowl and place the cornflakes in a third bowl.
4. Coat each scallop with the flour mixture, dip into the egg mixture and finally, dredge in the cornflakes.
5. Arrange scallops in the Air fryer basket and cook for about 6 minutes.
6. Dish out the scallops in a platter and serve hot.

- **Nutrition Info:** Calories: 150, Fat: 1.7g, Carbohydrates: 8g, Sugar: 0.4g, Protein: 24g, Sodium: 278mg

120.Sesame Mustard Greens

Servings: 4
Cooking Time: 11 Minutes

Ingredients:

- 2 garlic cloves, minced
- 1 pound mustard greens, torn
- 1 tablespoon olive oil
- ½ cup yellow onion, sliced
- Salt and black pepper to the taste
- 3 tablespoons veggie stock
- ¼ teaspoon dark sesame oil

Directions:

1. Heat up a pan that fits your air fryer with the oil over medium heat, add onions, stir and brown them for 5 minutes.
2. Add garlic, stock, greens, salt and pepper, stir, introduce in your air fryer and cook at 350 °F for 6 minutes.
3. Add sesame oil, toss to coat, divide among plates and serve.

- **Nutrition Info:** Calories: 173; Fat: 6g; Fiber: 2g; Carbs: 4g; Protein: 5g

121.Creamy Lemon Turkey

Servings: 4
Cooking Time: 20 Minutes

Ingredients:

- 1/3 cup sour cream
- 2 cloves garlic, finely minced 1/3 tsp. lemon zest
- 2 small-sized turkey breasts, skinless and cubed 1/3 cup thickened cream
- 2 tablespoons lemon juice
- 1 tsp. fresh marjoram, chopped
- Salt and freshly cracked mixed peppercorns, to taste 1/2 cup scallion, chopped
- 1/2 can tomatoes, diced
- 1½ tablespoons canola oil

Directions:

1. Firstly, pat dry the turkey breast. Mix the remaining items; marinate the turkey for 2 hours.

2. Set the air fryer to cook at 355 °F. Brush the turkey with a nonstick spray; cook for 23 minutes, turning once. Serve with naan and enjoy!

- **Nutrition Info:** 260 Calories; 15.3g Fat; 8.9g Carbs; 28.6g Protein; 1.9g Sugars

122.Bbq Pork Ribs

Servings: 2 To 3
Cooking Time: 5 Hrs 30 Minutes

Ingredients:

- 1 lb pork ribs
- 1 tsp soy sauce
- Salt and black pepper to taste
- 1 tsp oregano
- 1 tbsp + 1 tbsp maple syrup
- 3 tbsp barbecue sauce
- 2 cloves garlic, minced
- 1 tbsp cayenne pepper
- 1 tsp sesame oil

Directions:

1. Put the chops on a chopping board and use a knife to cut them into smaller pieces of desired sizes. Put them in a mixing bowl, add the soy sauce, salt, pepper, oregano, one tablespoon of maple syrup, barbecue sauce, garlic, cayenne pepper, and sesame oil. Mix well and place the pork in the fridge to marinate in the spices for 5 hours.
2. Preheat the Air Fryer to 350 F. Open the Air Fryer and place the ribs in the fryer basket. Slide the fryer basket in and cook for 15 minutes. Open the Air fryer, turn the ribs using tongs, apply the remaining maple syrup with a brush, close the Air Fryer, and continue cooking for 10 minutes.

- **Nutrition Info:** 346 Calories; 11g Fat; 4g Carbs; 32g Protein; 1g Sugars; 1g Fiber

123.Broccoli And Tomato Sauce

Servings: 4
Cooking Time: 7 Minutes

Ingredients:

- 1 broccoli head, florets separated
- ¼ cup scallions; chopped
- ½ cup tomato sauce
- 1 tbsp. olive oil
- 1 tbsp. sweet paprika
- Salt and black pepper to taste.

Directions:

1. In a pan that fits the air fryer, combine the broccoli with the rest of the Ingredients: toss.
2. Put the pan in the fryer and cook at 380°F for 15 minutes
3. Divide between plates and serve.

- **Nutrition Info:** Calories: 163; Fat: 5g; Fiber: 2g; Carbs: 4g; Protein: 8g

124.Paprika Crab Burgers

Servings: 3
Cooking Time: 20 Minutes

Ingredients:

- 2 eggs, beaten
- 1 shallot, chopped
- 2 garlic cloves, crushed
- 1 tablespoon olive oil
- 1 teaspoon yellow mustard
- 1 teaspoon fresh cilantro, chopped
- 10 ounces crab meat
- 1 teaspoon smoked paprika
- 1/2 teaspoon ground black pepper
- Sea salt, to taste
- 3/4 cup parmesan cheese

Directions:

1. In a mixing bowl, thoroughly combine the eggs, shallot, garlic, olive oil, mustard, cilantro, crab meat, paprika, black pepper, and salt. Mix until well combined.
2. Shape the mixture into 6 patties. Roll the crab patties over grated parmesan cheese, coating well on all sides. Place in your refrigerator for 2 hours.
3. Spritz the crab patties with cooking oil on both sides. Cook in the preheated Air Fryer at 360 degrees F for 14 minutes. Serve on dinner rolls if desired.

- **Nutrition Info:** 279 Calories; 14g Fat; 7g Carbs; 23g Protein; 5g Sugars; 6g Fiber

125.Cheese Zucchini Boats

Servings: 2
Cooking Time: 20 Minutes

Ingredients:

- 2 medium zucchinis
- ¼ cup full-fat ricotta cheese

- ¼ cup shredded mozzarella cheese
- ¼ cup low-carb, no-sugar-added pasta sauce.
- 2 tbsp. grated vegetarian Parmesan cheese
- 1 tbsp. avocado oil
- ¼ tsp. garlic powder.
- ½ tsp. dried parsley.
- ¼ tsp. dried oregano.

Directions:

1. Cut off 1-inch from the top and bottom of each zucchini.
2. Slice zucchini in half lengthwise and use a spoon to scoop out a bit of the inside, making room for filling. Brush with oil and spoon 2 tbsp. pasta sauce into each shell
3. Take a medium bowl, mix ricotta, mozzarella, oregano, garlic powder and parsley
4. Spoon the mixture into each zucchini shell. Place stuffed zucchini shells into the air fryer basket.
5. Adjust the temperature to 350 Degrees F and set the timer for 20 minutes
6. To remove from the fryer basket, use tongs or a spatula and carefully lift out. Top with Parmesan. Serve immediately.

- **Nutrition Info:** Calories: 215; Protein: 15g; Fiber: 7g; Fat: 19g; Carbs: 3g

126.Rice Flour Coated Shrimp

Servings: 3

Cooking Time: 20 Minutes

Ingredients:

- 3 tablespoons rice flour
- 1 pound shrimp, peeled and deveined
- 2 tablespoons olive oil
- 1 teaspoon powdered sugar
- Salt and black pepper, as required

Directions:

1. Preheat the Air fryer to 325 ºF and grease an Air fryer basket.
2. Mix rice flour, olive oil, sugar, salt, and black pepper in a bowl.
3. Stir in the shrimp and transfer half of the shrimp to the Air fryer basket.
4. Cook for about 10 minutes, flipping once in between.
5. Dish out the mixture onto serving plates and repeat with the remaining mixture.

- **Nutrition Info:** Calories: 299, Fat: 12g, Carbohydrates: 11.1g, Sugar: 0.8g, Protein: 35g, Sodium: 419mg

127.Marinated Cajun Beef

Servings: 2

Cooking Time: 20 Minutes

Ingredients:

- 1/3 cup beef broth
- 2 tablespoons Cajun seasoning, crushed
- 1/2 teaspoon garlic powder
- 3/4 pound beef tenderloins
- ½ tablespoon pear cider vinegar
- 1/3 teaspoon cayenne pepper
- 1 ½ tablespoon olive oil
- 1/2 teaspoon freshly ground black pepper
- 1 teaspoon salt

Directions:

1. Firstly, coat the beef tenderloins with salt, cayenne pepper, and black pepper.
2. Mix the remaining items in a medium-sized bowl; let the meat marinate for 40 minutes in this mixture.
3. Roast the beef for about 22 minutes at 385 degrees F, turning it halfway through the cooking time.

- **Nutrition Info:** 483 Calories; 23g Fat; 5g Carbs; 53g Protein; 6g Sugars; 4g Fiber

128.Buttered Scallops

Servings: 2

Cooking Time: 4 Minutes

Ingredients:

- ¾ pound sea scallops, cleaned and patted very dry
- 1 tablespoon butter, melted
- ½ tablespoon fresh thyme, minced
- Salt and black pepper, as required

Directions:

1. Preheat the Air fryer to 390 degree F and grease an Air fryer basket.
2. Mix scallops, butter, thyme, salt, and black pepper in a bowl.
3. Arrange scallops in the Air fryer basket and cook for about 4 minutes.

4. Dish out the scallops in a platter and serve hot.

- **Nutrition Info:** Calories: 202, Fat: 7.1g, Carbohydrates: 4.4g, Sugar: 0g, Protein: 28.7g, Sodium: 393mg

129.Okra With Green Beans

Servings: 2
Cooking Time: 20 Minutes
Ingredients:

- ½, 10-ouncesbag frozen cut okra
- ½, 10-ouncesbag frozen cut green beans
- ¼ cup nutritional yeast
- 3 tablespoons balsamic vinegar
- Salt and black pepper, to taste

Directions:

1. Preheat the Air fryer to 400 ºF and grease an Air fryer basket.
2. Mix the okra, green beans, nutritional yeast, vinegar, salt, and black pepper in a bowl and toss to coat well.
3. Arrange the okra mixture into the Air fryer basket and cook for about 20 minutes.
4. Dish out in a serving dish and serve hot.

- **Nutrition Info:** Calories: 126, Fat: 1.3g, Carbohydrates: 19.7g, Sugar: 2.1g, Protein: 11.9g, Sodium: 100mg

130.Korean Beef Bowl

Servings: 4
Cooking Time: 18 Minutes
Ingredients:

- 1 tablespoon minced garlic
- 1 teaspoon ground ginger
- 4 oz chive stems, chopped
- 2 tablespoon apple cider vinegar
- 1 teaspoon stevia extract
- 1 tablespoon flax seeds
- 1 teaspoon olive oil
- 1 teaspoon olive oil
- 1-pound ground beef
- 4 tablespoon chicken stock

Directions:

1. Sprinkle the ground beef with the apple cider vinegar and stir the meat with the help of the spoon.
2. After this, sprinkle the ground beef with the ground ginger, minced garlic, and olive oil.
3. Mix it up.
4. Preheat the air fryer to 370 F.
5. Put the ground beef in the air fryer basket tray and cook it for 8 minutes.
6. After this, stir the ground beef carefully and sprinkle with the chopped chives, flax seeds, olive oil, and chicken stock.
7. Mix the dish up and cook it for 10 minutes more.
8. When the time is over - stir the dish carefully.
9. Serve Korean beef bowl immediately.
10. Enjoy!

- **Nutrition Info:** calories 258, fat 10.1, fiber 1.2, carbs 4.2, protein 35.3

131.Garlic Lamb Shank

Servings: 5
Cooking Time: 24 Minutes
Ingredients:

- 17 oz. lamb shanks
- 2 tablespoon garlic, peeled
- 1 teaspoon kosher salt
- 1 tablespoon dried parsley
- 4 oz chive stems, chopped
- ½ cup chicken stock
- 1 teaspoon butter
- 1 teaspoon dried rosemary
- 1 teaspoon nutmeg
- ½ teaspoon ground black pepper

Directions:

1. Chop the garlic roughly.
2. Make the cuts in the lamb shank and fill the cuts with the chopped garlic.
3. Then sprinkle the lamb shank with the kosher salt, dried parsley, dried rosemary, nutmeg, and ground black pepper.
4. Stir the spices on the lamb shank gently.
5. Then put the butter and chicken stock in the air fryer basket tray.
6. Preheat the air fryer to 380 F.
7. Put the chives in the air fryer basket tray.
8. Add the lamb shank and cook the meat for 24 minutes.
9. When the lamb shank is cooked - transfer it to the serving plate and sprinkle with the remaining liquid from the cooked meat.
10. Enjoy!

- **Nutrition Info:** calories 205, fat 8.2, fiber 0.8, carbs 3.8, protein 27.2

132.Chinese-style Spicy And Herby Beef

Servings: 4
Cooking Time: 20 Minutes
Ingredients:

- 1 pound flank steak, cut into small pieces
- 1 teaspoon fresh sage leaves, minced
- 1/3 cup olive oil
- 3 teaspoons sesame oil
- 3 tablespoons Shaoxing wine
- 2 tablespoons tamari
- 1 teaspoon hot sauce
- 1/8 teaspoon xanthum gum
- 1 teaspoon seasoned salt
- 3 cloves garlic,minced
- 1 teaspoon fresh rosemary leaves, finely minced
- 1/2 teaspoon freshly cracked black pepper

Directions:

1. Warm the oil in a sauté pan over a moderate heat. Now, sauté the garlic until just tender and fragrant.
2. Now, add the remaining ingredients. Toss to coat well.
3. Then, roast for about 18 minutes at 345 degrees F. Check doneness and serve warm.

- **Nutrition Info:** 354 Calories; 24g Fat; 8g Carbs; 21g Protein; 3g Sugars; 3g Fiber

133.Dinner Avocado Chicken Sliders

Servings: 4
Cooking Time: 20 Minutes
Ingredients:

- ½ pounds ground chicken meat 4 burger buns
- 1/2 cup Romaine lettuce, loosely packed
- ½ tsp. dried parsley flakes 1/3 tsp. mustard seeds
- 1 tsp. onion powder
- 1 ripe fresh avocado, mashed 1 tsp. garlic powder
- 1 ½ tablespoon extra-virgin olive oil
- 1 cloves garlic, minced Nonstick cooking spray
- Salt and cracked black pepper (peppercorns, to taste)

Directions:

1. Firstly, spritz an air fryer cooking basket with a nonstick cooking spray.
2. Mix ground chicken meat, mustard seeds, garlic powder, onion powder, parsley, salt, and black pepper until everything is thoroughly combined. Make sure not to overwork the meat to avoid tough chicken burgers.
3. Shape the meat mixture into patties and roll them in breadcrumbs; transfer your burgers to the prepared cooking basket. Brush the patties with the cooking spray.
4. Air-fry at 355 F for 9 minutes, working in batches. Slice burger buns into halves. In the meantime, combine olive oil with mashed avocado and pressed garlic.
5. To finish, lay Romaine lettuce and avocado spread on bun bottoms; now, add burgers and bun tops.

- **Nutrition Info:** 321 Calories; 18.7g Fat; 15.8g Carbs; 1.2g Sugars

134.Flank Steak Beef

Servings: 4
Cooking Time: 20 Minutes
Ingredients:

- 1 pound flank steaks, sliced
- ¼ cup xanthum gum
- 2 teaspoon vegetable oil
- ½ teaspoon ginger
- ½ cup soy sauce
- 1 tablespoon garlic, minced
- ½ cup water
- ¾ cup swerve, packed

Directions:

1. Preheat the Air fryer to 390 degree F and grease an Air fryer basket.
2. Coat the steaks with xanthum gum on both the sides and transfer into the Air fryer basket.
3. Cook for about 10 minutes and dish out in a platter.
4. Meanwhile, cook rest of the ingredients for the sauce in a saucepan.
5. Bring to a boil and pour over the steak slices to serve.

- **Nutrition Info:** Calories: 372, Fat: 11.8g, Carbohydrates: 1.8g, Sugar: 27.3g, Protein: 34g, Sodium: 871mg

135.Traditional English Fish And Chips

Servings: 4
Cooking Time: 17 Minutes
Ingredients:

- 1 3/4 pounds potatoes
- 4 tablespoons olive oil
- 1-1/4 teaspoons kosher salt
- 1-1/4 teaspoons black pepper
- 8 sprigs fresh thyme
- 4 (6-ounce) pieces cod
- 1 lemon
- 1 clove garlic
- 2 tablespoons capers

Directions:

1. Start by preheating toaster oven to 450°F.
2. Cut potatoes into 1-inch chunks.
3. Place potatoes, 2 tablespoons oil, salt, and thyme in a baking tray and toss to combine.
4. Spread in a flat layer and bake for 30 minutes.
5. Wrap mixture in foil to keep warm.
6. Wipe tray with a paper towel and then lay cod in the tray.
7. Slice the lemon and top cod with lemon, salt, pepper, and thyme.
8. Drizzle rest of the oil over the cod and bake for 12 minutes.
9. Place cod and potatoes on separate pans and bake together for an additional 5 minutes.
10. Combine and serve.

- **Nutrition Info:** Calories: 442, Sodium: 1002 mg, Dietary Fiber: 5.4 g, Total Fat: 15.8 g, Total Carbs: 32.7 g, Protein: 42.5 g.

136.Smoked Sausage And Bacon Shashlik

Servings: 4
Cooking Time: 20 Minutes
Ingredients:

- 1 pound smoked Polish beef sausage, sliced
- 1 tablespoon mustard
- 1 tablespoon olive oil
- 2 tablespoons Worcestershire sauce
- 2 bell peppers, sliced
- Salt and ground black pepper, to taste

Directions:

1. Toss the sausage with the mustard, olive, and Worcestershire sauce. Thread sausage and peppers onto skewers.
2. Sprinkle with salt and black pepper.
3. Cook in the preheated Air Fryer at 360 degrees Ffor 11 minutes. Brush the skewers with the reserved marinade.

- **Nutrition Info:** 422 Calories; 36g Fat; 9g Carbs; 18g Protein; 6g Sugars; 7g Fiber

137.Turkey Wontons With Garlic-parmesan Sauce

Servings: 8
Cooking Time: 20 Minutes
Ingredients:

- 8 ounces cooked turkey breasts, shredded 16 wonton wrappers
- 1½ tablespoons margarine, melted
- 1/3 cup cream cheese, room temperature 8 ounces Asiago cheese, shredded
- 3 tablespoons Parmesan cheese, grated
- 1 tsp. garlic powder
- Fine sea salt and freshly ground black pepper, to taste

Directions:

1. In a small-sized bowl, mix the margarine, Parmesan, garlic powder, salt, and black pepper; give it a good stir.
2. Lightly grease a mini muffin pan; lay 1 wonton wrapper in each mini muffin cup. Fill each cup with the cream cheese and turkey mixture.
3. Air-fry for 8 minutes at 335 °F. Immediately top with Asiago cheese and serve warm.

- **Nutrition Info:** 362 Calories; 13.5g Fat; 40.4g Carbs; 18.5g Protein; 1.2g Sugars

138.Tomato Stuffed Pork Roll

Servings: 4
Cooking Time: 15 Minutes
Ingredients:

- 1 scallion, chopped
- ¼ cup sun-dried tomatoes, chopped finely
- 2 tablespoons fresh parsley, chopped
- 4: 6-ouncepork cutlets, pounded slightly

- Salt and freshly ground black pepper, to taste
- 2 teaspoons paprika
- ½ tablespoon olive oil

Directions:

1. Preheat the Air fryer to 390 degree F and grease an Air fryer basket.
2. Mix scallion, tomatoes, parsley, salt and black pepper in a bowl.
3. Coat each cutlet with tomato mixture and roll up the cutlet, securing with cocktail sticks.
4. Coat the rolls with oil and rub with paprika, salt and black pepper.
5. Arrange the rolls in the Air fryer basket and cook for about 15 minutes, flipping once in between.
6. Dish out in a platter and serve warm.

- **Nutrition Info:** Calories: 244, Fat: 14.5g, Carbohydrates: 20.1g, Sugar: 1.7g, Protein: 8.2g, Sodium: 670mg

139.Zucchini Muffins

Servings: 8
Cooking Time: 20 Minutes
Ingredients:

- 6 eggs
- 4 drops stevia 1/4 cup Swerve
- 1/3 cup coconut oil, melted 1 cup zucchini, grated
- 3/4 cup coconut flour 1/4 tsp ground nutmeg 1 tsp ground cinnamon 1/2 tsp baking soda

Directions:

1. Preheat the air fryer to 325 F.
2. Add all ingredients except zucchini in a bowl and mix well.
3. Add zucchini and stir well.
4. Pour batter into the silicone muffin molds and place into the air fryer basket.
5. Cook muffins for 20 minutes.
6. Serve and enjoy.

- **Nutrition Info:** Calories 136 Fat 12 g Carbohydrates 1 g Sugar 0.6 g Protein 4 g Cholesterol 123 mg

140.Beef, Olives And Tomatoes

Servings: 4
Cooking Time: 35 Minutes
Ingredients:

- 2pounds beef stew meat, cubed
- 1cup black olives, pitted and halved
- 1cup cherry tomatoes, halved
- 1tablespoon smoked paprika
- 3tablespoons olive oil
- 1teaspoon coriander, ground
- Salt and black pepper to the taste

Directions:

1. In the air fryer's pan, mix the beef with the olives and the other ingredients, toss and cook at 390 degrees F for 35 minutes.
2. Divide between plates and serve.

- **Nutrition Info:** Calories 291, Fat 12, Fiber 9, Carbs 20, Protein 26

141.Healthy Mama Meatloaf

Servings: 8
Cooking Time: 40 Minutes
Ingredients:

- 1 tablespoon olive oil
- 1 green bell pepper, diced
- 1/2 cup diced sweet onion
- 1/2 teaspoon minced garlic
- 1-lb. ground beef
- 1 cup whole wheat bread crumbs
- 2 large eggs
- 3/4 cup shredded carrot
- 3/4 cup shredded zucchini
- salt and ground black pepper to taste
- 1/4 cup ketchup, or to taste

Directions:

1. Thoroughly mix ground beef with egg, onion, garlic, crumbs, and all the ingredients in a bowl.
2. Grease a meatloaf pan with oil or butter and spread the minced beef in the pan.
3. Press "Power Button" of Air Fry Oven and turn the dial to select the "Bake" mode.
4. Press the Time button and again turn the dial to set the cooking time to 40 minutes.
5. Now push the Temp button and rotate the dial to set the temperature at 375 degrees F.
6. Once preheated, place the beef baking pan in the oven and close its lid.
7. Slice and serve.

- **Nutrition Info:** Calories: 322 Cal Total Fat: 11.8 g Saturated Fat: 2.2 g Cholesterol: 56 mg Sodium: 321 mg Total Carbs: 14.6 g Fiber: 4.4 g Sugar: 8 g Protein: 17.3 g

142.Air Fryer Roasted Broccoli

Servings: 4
Cooking Time: 10 Minutes
Ingredients:

- 1 tsp. herbes de provence seasoning (optional)
- 4 cups fresh broccoli
- 1 tablespoon olive oil
- Salt and pepper to taste

Directions:

1. Drizzle or spray broccoli with olive and sprinkle seasoning throughout
2. Spray air fryer basket with cooking oil, place broccoli and cook for 5-8 minutes on 360F
3. Open air fryer and examine broccoli after 5 minutes because different fryer brands cook at different rates.

- **Nutrition Info:** Calories 61 Fat 4g protein 3g net carbs 4g

143.Morning Ham And Cheese Sandwich

Servings: 4
Cooking Time: 15 Minutes
Ingredients:

- 8 slices whole wheat bread
- 4 slices lean pork ham
- 4 slices cheese
- 8 slices tomato

Directions:

1. Preheat your air fryer to 360 f. Lay four slices of bread on a flat surface. Spread the slices with cheese, tomato, turkey and ham. Cover with the remaining slices to form sandwiches. Add the sandwiches to the air fryer cooking basket and cook for 10 minutes.

- **Nutrition Info:** Calories: 361 Cal Total Fat: 16.7 g Saturated Fat: 0 g Cholesterol: 0 mg Sodium: 1320 mg Total Carbs: 32.5 g Fiber: 2.3 g Sugar: 5.13 g Protein: 19.3 g

144.Stuffed Potatoes

Servings: 4
Cooking Time: 31 Minutes
Ingredients:

- 4 potatoes, peeled
- 1 tablespoon butter
- ½ of brown onion, chopped
- 2 tablespoons chives, chopped
- ½ cup Parmesan cheese, grated
- 3 tablespoons canola oil

Directions:

1. Preheat the Air fryer to 390 ºF and grease an Air fryer basket.
2. Coat the potatoes with canola oil and arrange into the Air fryer basket.
3. Cook for about 20 minutes and transfer into a platter.
4. Cut each potato in half and scoop out the flesh from each half.
5. Heat butter in a frying pan over medium heat and add onions.
6. Sauté for about 5 minutes and dish out in a bowl.
7. Mix the onions with the potato flesh, chives, and half of cheese.
8. Stir well and stuff the potato halves evenly with the onion potato mixture.
9. Top with the remaining cheese and arrange the potato halves into the Air fryer basket.
10. Cook for about 6 minutes and dish out to serve warm.

- **Nutrition Info:** Calories: 328, Fat: 11.3g, Carbohydrates: 34.8g, Sugar: 3.1g, Protein: 5.8g, Sodium: 77mg

145.Chili Pepper Lamb Chops

Servings: 6
Cooking Time: 10 Minutes
Ingredients:

- 21 oz. lamb chops
- 1 teaspoon chili pepper
- ½ teaspoon chili flakes
- 1 teaspoon onion powder
- 1 teaspoon garlic powder
- 1 teaspoon cayenne pepper
- 1 tablespoon olive oil
- 1 tablespoon butter

- ½ teaspoon lime zest

Directions:

1. Melt the butter and combine it with the olive oil.
2. Whisk the liquid and add chili pepper, chili flakes, onion powder, garlic powder, cayenne pepper, and lime zest.
3. Whisk it well
4. Then sprinkle the lamb chops with the prepared oily marinade.
5. Leave the meat for at least 5 minutes in the fridge.
6. Preheat the air fryer to 400 F.
7. Place the marinated lamb chops in the air fryer and cook them for 5 minutes.
8. After this, open the air fryer and turn the lamb chops into another side.
9. Cook the lamb chops for 5 minutes more.
10. When the meat is cooked – transfer it to the serving plates.
11. Enjoy!

- **Nutrition Info:** calories 227, fat 11.6, fiber 0.2, carbs 1, protein 28.1

146.Spicy Paprika Steak

Servings: 2
Cooking Time: 20 Minutes
Ingredients:

- 1/2 Ancho chili pepper, soaked in hot water before using
- 1 tablespoon brandy
- 2 teaspoons smoked paprika
- 1 1/2 tablespoons olive oil
- 2 beef steaks
- Kosher salt, to taste
- 1 teaspoon ground allspice
- 3 cloves garlic, sliced

Directions:

1. Sprinkle the beef steaks with salt, paprika, and allspice. Add the steak to a baking dish that fits your fryer. Scatter the sliced garlic over the top.
2. Now, drizzle it with brandy and olive oil; spread minced Ancho chili pepper over the top.
3. Bake at 385 degrees F for 14 minutes, turning halfway through. Serve warm.

- **Nutrition Info:** 450 Calories; 26g Fat; 4g Carbs; 58g Protein; 3g Sugars; 3g Fiber

147.Steak With Cascabel-garlic Sauce

Servings: 4
Cooking Time: 20 Minutes
Ingredients:

- 2 teaspoons brown mustard
- 2 tablespoons mayonnaise
- 1 ½ pounds beef flank steak, trimmed and cubed
- 2 teaspoons minced cascabel
- ½ cup scallions, finely chopped
- 1/3 cup Crème fraîche
- 2 teaspoons cumin seeds
- 3 cloves garlic, pressed
- Pink peppercorns to taste, freshly cracked
- 1 teaspoon fine table salt
- 1/3 teaspoon black pepper, preferably freshly ground

Directions:

1. Firstly, fry the cumin seeds just about 1 minute or until they pop.
2. After that, season your beef flank steak with fine table salt, black pepper and the fried cumin seeds; arrange the seasoned beef cubes on the bottom of your baking dish that fits in the air fryer.
3. Throw in the minced cascabel, garlic, and scallions; air-fry approximately 8 minutes at 390 degrees F.
4. Once the beef cubes start to tender, add your favorite mayo, Crème fraîche, freshly cracked pink peppercorns and mustard; air-fry 7 minutes longer. Serve over hot wild rice.

- **Nutrition Info:** 329 Calories; 16g Fat; 8g Carbs; 37g Protein; 9g Sugars; 6g Fiber

148.Spicy Sesame-honey Chicken

Servings: 4
Cooking Time: 30 Minutes
Ingredients:

- 1 package of chicken thighs/wings
- 1 tablespoon sugar
- 1-1/3 tablespoons chili garlic sauce
- 1/4 cup soy sauce
- 1 tablespoon sesame oil

- 1 tablespoon ketchup
- 1 tablespoon honey
- 1 tablespoon soy sauce
- 1 teaspoon sugar or brown sugar
- 1 teaspoon cornstarch

Directions:

1. Create marinade by combining 1 tablespoon chili sauce, soy sauce, and sesame oil.
2. Toss chicken in marinade and refrigerate for at least 30 minutes, but up to a day.
3. Preheat toaster oven to 375°F. Place chicken on a baking sheet with a little space between each piece and bake for 30 minutes.
4. While the chicken bakes, create the sauce by combining all the leftover ingredients, including the 1/3 tablespoon of chili sauce.
5. Mix well and microwave in 30-second intervals until the sauce starts to thicken.
6. Toss chicken in sauce and serve.

- **Nutrition Info:** Calories: 401, Sodium: 1439 mg, Dietary Fiber: 0 g, Total Fat: 16.0 g, Total Carbs: 11.2 g, Protein: 50.6 g.

149.Pepper Pork Chops

Servings: 2
Cooking Time: 6 Minutes
Ingredients:

- 2 pork chops
- 1 egg white
- ¾ cup xanthum gum
- ½ teaspoon sea salt
- ¼ teaspoon freshly ground black pepper
- 1 oil mister

Directions:

1. Preheat the Air fryer to 400 degree F and grease an Air fryer basket.
2. Whisk egg white with salt and black pepper in a bowl and dip the pork chops in it.
3. Cover the bowl and marinate for about 20 minutes.
4. Pour the xanthum gum over both sides of the chops and spray with oil mister.
5. Arrange the chops in the Air fryer basket and cook for about 6 minutes.
6. Dish out in a bowl and serve warm.

- **Nutrition Info:** Calories: 541, Fat: 34g, Carbohydrates: 3.4g, Sugar: 1g, Protein: 20.3g, Sodium: 547mg

150.Garlic Butter Pork Chops

Servings: 4
Cooking Time: 8 Minutes
Ingredients:

- 4 pork chops
- 1 tablespoon coconut butter
- 2 teaspoons parsley
- 1 tablespoon coconut oil
- 2 teaspoons garlic, grated
- Salt and black pepper, to taste

Directions:

1. Preheat the Air fryer to 350 degree F and grease an Air fryer basket.
2. Mix all the seasonings, coconut oil, garlic, butter, and parsley in a bowl and coat the pork chops with it.
3. Cover the chops with foil and refrigerate to marinate for about 1 hour.
4. Remove the foil and arrange the chops in the Air fryer basket.
5. Cook for about 8 minutes and dish out in a bowl to serve warm.

- **Nutrition Info:** Calories: 311, Fat: 25.5g, Carbohydrates: 1.4g, Sugar: 0.3g, Protein: 18.4g, Sodium: 58mg

151.Sage Beef

Servings: 4
Cooking Time: 30 Minutes
Ingredients:

- 2pounds beef stew meat, cubed
- 1tablespoon sage, chopped
- 2tablespoons butter, melted
- ½ teaspoon coriander, ground
- ½ tablespoon garlic powder
- 1teaspoon Italian seasoning
- Salt and black pepper to the taste

Directions:

1. In the air fryer's pan, mix the beef with the sage, melted butter and the other ingredients, introduce the pan in the fryer and cook at 360 degrees F for 30 minutes.
2. Divide everything between plates and serve.

- **Nutrition Info:** Calories 290, Fat 11, Fiber 6, Carbs 20, Protein 29

152.Broccoli With Olives

Servings: 4
Cooking Time: 19 Minutes
Ingredients:

- 2 pounds broccoli, stemmed and cut into 1-inch florets
- 1/3 cup Kalamata olives, halved and pitted
- ¼ cup Parmesan cheese, grated
- 2 tablespoons olive oil
- Salt and ground black pepper, as required
- 2 teaspoons fresh lemon zest, grated

Directions:

1. Preheat the Air fryer to 400 ºF and grease an Air fryer basket.
2. Boil the broccoli for about 4 minutes and drain well.
3. Mix broccoli, oil, salt, and black pepper in a bowl and toss to coat well.
4. Arrange broccoli into the Air fryer basket and cook for about 15 minutes.
5. Stir in the olives, lemon zest and cheese and dish out to serve.

- **Nutrition Info:** Calories: 169, Fat: 10.2g, Carbohydrates: 16g, Sugar: 3.9g, Protein: 8.5g, Sodium: 254mg

153.Five Spice Pork

Servings: 4
Cooking Time: 20 Minutes
Ingredients:

- 1-pound pork belly
- 2 tablespoons swerve
- 2 tablespoons dark soy sauce
- 1 tablespoon Shaoxing: cooking wine
- 2 teaspoons garlic, minced
- 2 teaspoons ginger, minced
- 1 tablespoon hoisin sauce
- 1 teaspoon Chinese Five Spice

Directions:

1. Preheat the Air fryer to 390 degree F and grease an Air fryer basket.
2. Mix all the ingredients in a bowl and place in the Ziplock bag.
3. Seal the bag, shake it well and refrigerate to marinate for about 1 hour.
4. Remove the pork from the bag and arrange it in the Air fryer basket.
5. Cook for about 15 minutes and dish out in a bowl to serve warm.

- **Nutrition Info:** Calories: 604, Fat: 30.6g, Carbohydrates: 1.4g, Sugar: 20.3g, Protein: 19.8g, Sodium: 834mg

154.Spiced Salmon Kebabs

Servings: 3
Cooking Time: 15 Minutes
Ingredients:

- 2 tablespoons chopped fresh oregano
- 2 teaspoons sesame seeds
- 1 teaspoon ground cumin
- Salt and pepper to taste
- 1 ½ pounds salmon fillets
- 2 tablespoons olive oil
- 2 lemons, sliced into rounds

Directions:

1. Place the instant pot air fryer lid on and preheat the instant pot at 390 degrees F.
2. Place the grill pan accessory in the instant pot.
3. Create dry rub by combining the oregano, sesame seeds, cumin, salt, and pepper.
4. Rub the salmon fillets with the dry rub and brush with oil.
5. Place on the grill pan, close the air fryer lid and grill the salmon for 15 minutes.
6. Serve with lemon slices once cooked.

- **Nutrition Info:** Calories per serving 447 ; Carbs: 4.1g; Protein:47.6 g; Fat:26.6 g

155.Cheesy Shrimp

Servings: 4
Cooking Time: 20 Minutes
Ingredients:

- 2/3 cup Parmesan cheese, grated
- 2 pounds shrimp, peeled and deveined
- 4 garlic cloves, minced
- 2 tablespoons olive oil
- 1 teaspoon dried basil
- ½ teaspoon dried oregano
- 1 teaspoon onion powder
- ½ teaspoon red pepper flakes, crushed
- Ground black pepper, as required
- 2 tablespoons fresh lemon juice

Directions:

1. Preheat the Air fryer to 350 degree F and grease an Air fryer basket.
2. Mix Parmesan cheese, garlic, olive oil, herbs, and spices in a large bowl.
3. Arrange half of the shrimp into the Air fryer basket in a single layer and cook for about 10 minutes.
4. Dish out the shrimps onto serving plates and drizzle with lemon juice to serve hot.

- **Nutrition Info:** Calories: 386, Fat: 14.2g, Carbohydrates: 5.3g, Sugar: 0.4g, Protein: 57.3g, Sodium: 670mg

156.Salmon Casserole

Servings: 8

Cooking Time: 12 Minutes

Ingredients:

- 7 oz Cheddar cheese, shredded
- ½ cup cream
- 1-pound salmon fillet
- 1 tablespoon dried dill
- 1 teaspoon dried parsley
- 1 teaspoon salt
- 1 teaspoon ground coriander
- ½ teaspoon ground black pepper
- 2 green pepper, chopped
- 4 oz chive stems, diced
- 7 oz bok choy, chopped
- 1 tablespoon olive oil

Directions:

1. Sprinkle the salmon fillet with the dried dill, dried parsley, ground coriander, and ground black pepper.
2. Massage the salmon fillet gently and leave it for 5 minutes to make the fish soaks the spices.
3. Meanwhile, sprinkle the air fryer casserole tray with the olive oil inside.
4. After this, cut the salmon fillet into the cubes.
5. Separate the salmon cubes into 2 parts.
6. Then place the first part of the salmon cubes in the casserole tray.
7. Sprinkle the fish with the chopped bok choy, diced chives, and chopped green pepper.
8. After this, place the second part of the salmon cubes over the vegetables.
9. Then sprinkle the casserole with the shredded cheese and heavy cream.
10. Preheat the air fryer to 380 F.
11. Cook the salmon casserole for 12 minutes.
12. When the dish is cooked – it will have acrunchy light brown crust.
13. Serve it and enjoy!

- **Nutrition Info:** calories 216, fat 14.4, fiber 1.1, carbs 4.3, protein 18.2

MEAT RECIPES

157.Steak Seasoned Pork Chops

Servings: 4
Cooking Time: 12 Minutes
Ingredients:

- 1 lb pork chops, boneless
- 1 tsp steak seasoning blend
- 1 tbsp yellow mustard
- 2 tsp honey

Directions:

1. Fit the oven with the rack in position 2.
2. Line the air fryer basket with parchment paper.
3. In a small bowl, mix honey, mustard, and steak seasoning.
4. Brush pork chops with honey mixture and place in air fryer basket then place air fryer basket in baking pan.
5. Place a baking pan on the oven rack. Set to air fry at 350 F for 12 minutes.
6. Serve and enjoy.

- **Nutrition Info:** Calories 376 Fat 28.3 g Carbohydrates 3.1 g Sugar 2.9 g Protein 25.7 g Cholesterol 98 mg

158.Meatballs(3)

Servings: 4
Cooking Time: 20 Minutes
Ingredients:

- 1 lb ground beef
- 1/2 small onion, chopped
- 1 egg, lightly beaten
- 2 garlic cloves, minced
- 1 tbsp basil, chopped
- 1/4 cup parmesan cheese, grated
- 1/2 cup breadcrumbs
- 1 tbsp Italian parsley, chopped
- 1 tbsp rosemary, chopped
- 2 tbsp milk
- Pepper
- Salt

Directions:

1. Fit the oven with the rack in position
2. Add all ingredients into the mixing bowl and mix until well combined.
3. Make small balls from the meat mixture and place them into the baking pan.
4. Set to bake at 375 F for 25 minutes. After 5 minutes place the baking pan in the preheated oven.
5. Serve and enjoy.

- **Nutrition Info:** Calories 311 Fat 10.4 g Carbohydrates 12.3 g Sugar 1.7 g Protein 39.9 g Cholesterol 147 mg

159.Baked Spinach Cheese Chicken

Servings: 2
Cooking Time: 20 Minutes
Ingredients:

- 2 chicken breasts, boneless & skinless
- 1/2 tsp garlic powder
- 1/4 cup sun-dried tomatoes, chopped
- 1/4 cup cheddar cheese, shredded
- 3 oz cream cheese
- 2 cups fresh spinach, chopped
- 3/4 tsp pepper
- 3/4 tsp salt

Directions:

1. Fit the oven with the rack in position
2. Slice the chicken breasts into the half and place them into the baking dish. Season with pepper and salt.
3. Cook spinach in the pan until wilted.
4. In a bowl, mix spinach, garlic powder, tomatoes, cheddar cheese, and cream cheese.
5. Spread spinach mixture on top of chicken breasts.
6. Set to bake at 425 F for 25 minutes. After 5 minutes place the baking dish in the preheated oven.
7. Serve and enjoy.

- **Nutrition Info:** Calories 498 Fat 30.5 g Carbohydrates 4.3 g Sugar 1.1 g Protein 50.2 g Cholesterol 192 mg

160.Chicken With Potatoes And Corn

Servings:4
Cooking Time: 25 Minutes
Ingredients:

- 4 bone-in, skin-on chicken thighs
- 2 teaspoons kosher salt, divided

- 1 cup Bisquick baking mix
- ½ cup butter, melted, divided
- 1 pound (454 g) small red potatoes, quartered
- 3 ears corn, shucked and cut into rounds 1- to 1½-inches thick
- $^1/_3$ cup heavy whipping cream
- ½ teaspoon freshly ground black pepper

Directions:

1. Sprinkle the chicken on all sides with 1 teaspoon of kosher salt. Place the baking mix in a shallow dish. Brush the thighs on all sides with ¼ cup of butter, then dredge them in the baking mix, coating them all on sides. Place the chicken in the center of the baking pan.
2. Place the potatoes in a large bowl with 2 tablespoons of butter and toss to coat. Place them on one side of the chicken on the pan.
3. Place the corn in a medium bowl and drizzle with the remaining butter. Sprinkle with ¼ teaspoon of kosher salt and toss to coat. Place on the pan on the other side of the chicken.
4. Slide the baking pan into Rack Position 2, select Roast, set temperature to 375ºF (190ºC), and set time to 25 minutes.
5. After 20 minutes, remove from the oven and put the potatoes back to the bowl. Return the pan to oven and continue cooking.
6. As the chicken continues cooking, add the cream, black pepper, and remaining kosher salt to the potatoes. Lightly mash the potatoes with a potato masher.
7. When cooking is complete, the corn should be tender and the chicken cooked through, reading 165ºF (74ºC) on a meat thermometer. Remove from the oven. Serve the chicken with the smashed potatoes and corn on the side.

161.Beef Flat Cakes

Servings:x

Cooking Time:x

Ingredients:

- 2 tbsp. garam masala
- 1 lb. sliced beef steak
- 3 tsp ginger finely chopped
- 1-2 tbsp. fresh coriander leaves
- 2 or 3 green chilies finely chopped
- 1 ½ tbsp. lemon juice
- Salt and pepper to taste

Directions:

1. Mix the ingredients in a clean bowl and add water to it. Make sure that the paste is not too watery but is enough to apply on the sides of the steak. Pre heat the oven at 160 degrees Fahrenheit for 5 minutes.
2. Place the French Cuisine Galettes in the fry basket and let them cook for another 25 minutes at the same temperature. Keep rolling them over to get a uniform cook. Serve either with mint sauce or ketchup.

162.Copycat Chicken Sandwich

Servings: 4

Cooking Time: 15 Minutes

Ingredients:

- 2 chicken breasts, boneless & skinless
- 1 cup buttermilk
- 1 tbsp. + 2 tsp paprika, divided
- 1 tbsp. + 1 ½ tsp garlic powder, divided
- 2 tsp salt, divided
- 2 tsp pepper, divided
- 4 brioche buns
- 1 cup flour
- ½ cup corn starch
- 1 tbsp. onion powder
- 1 tbsp. cayenne pepper
- ½ cup mayonnaise
- 1 tsp hot sauce
- Sliced pickles

Directions:

1. Place chicken between two sheets of plastic wrap and pound to ½-inch thick. Cut crosswise to get 4 cutlets.
2. In a large bowl, whisk together buttermilk and one teaspoon each paprika, garlic powder, salt, and pepper. Add chicken, cover, and refrigerate overnight.
3. Place the buns on the baking pan and place in position 2 of the oven. Set to toast for about 2-5 minutes depending how toasted you want them. Set aside.

4. In a medium shallow dish, combine flour, cornstarch, onion powder, cayenne pepper, and remaining paprika, garlic powder, salt, and pepper.
5. Whisk in 2-3 tablespoons of the buttermilk batter chicken was marinating in until smooth.
6. Lightly spray fryer basket with cooking spray.
7. Dredge chicken in the flour mixture forming a thick coating of the batter. Place in fryer basket.
8. Place basket in the oven. Set oven to air fryer on 375°F for 10 minutes. Cook until crispy and golden brown, turning chicken over halfway through cooking time.
9. In a small bowl, whisk together mayonnaise, hot sauce, 1 teaspoon paprika, and ½ teaspoon garlic powder.
10. To serve, spread top of buns with mayonnaise mixture. Place chicken on bottom buns and top with pickles then top bun.

- **Nutrition Info:** Calories 689, Total Fat 27g, Saturated Fat 5g, Total Carbs 71g, Net Carbs 67g, Protein 38g, Sugar 7g, Fiber 4g, Sodium 1734mg, Potassium 779mg, Phosphorus 435mg

163.Chili Chicken Strips With Aioli

Servings:4
Cooking Time: 20 Minutes
Ingredients:

- 1 lb chicken breasts, cut into strips
- 2 tbsp olive oil
- 1 cup breadcrumbs
- ½ tbsp garlic powder
- ½ tbsp chili powder
- ½ cup mayonnaise

Directions:

1. Preheat on AirFry function to 350 F. Mix breadcrumbs, garlic powder, and chili in a plate. Coat the strips in the breadcrumb mixture. Drizzle with olive oil.
2. Arrange the chicken strips on the basket and press Start. Cook for 12-14 minutes. To prepare the aioli: combine mayo with ground chili. Serve with the chicken strips.

164.Garlic Lemony Chicken Breast

Servings:2
Cooking Time: 20 Minutes
Ingredients:

- 1 chicken breast
- 2 lemon, juiced and rind reserved
- 1 tbsp chicken seasoning
- 1 tbsp garlic puree
- A handful of peppercorns
- Salt and black pepper to taste

Directions:

1. Place a silver foil sheet on a flat surface. Add all seasonings alongside the lemon rind. Lay the chicken breast onto a chopping board and trim any fat and little bones; season.
2. Rub the chicken seasoning on both sides. Place on the foil sheet and seal tightly; flatten with a rolling pin. Place the breast in the basket and cook for 15 minutes at 350 F on AirFry function.

165.Cheesy Pepperoni And Chicken Pizza

Servings:6
Cooking Time: 15 Minutes
Ingredients:

- 2 cups cooked chicken, cubed
- 1 cup pizza sauce
- 20 slices pepperoni
- ¼ cup grated Parmesan cheese
- 1 cup shredded Mozzarella cheese
- Cooking spray

Directions:

1. Spritz the baking pan with cooking spray.
2. Arrange the chicken cubes in the prepared baking pan, then top the cubes with pizza sauce and pepperoni. Stir to coat the cubes and pepperoni with sauce. Scatter the cheeses on top.
3. Put the air fryer basket on the baking pan and slide into Rack Position 2, select Air Fry, set temperature to 375ºF (190ºC) and set time to 15 minutes.
4. When cooking is complete, the pizza should be frothy and the cheeses should be melted.
5. Serve immediately.

166.Sweet Asian Chicken Wings

Servings:4

Cooking Time: 25 Minutes

Ingredients:

- 1 lb chicken wings
- 1 cup flour
- 1 cup breadcrumbs
- 2 eggs, beaten
- 2 tbsp canola oil
- Salt and black pepper to taste
- 2 tbsp sesame seeds
- 2 tbsp Korean red pepper paste
- 1 tbsp apple cider vinegar
- 2 tbsp honey
- 1 tbsp soy sauce

Directions:

1. Preheat on AirFry function to 390 F. Separate the chicken wings into winglets and drumettes. In a bowl, mix oil, salt, and pepper. Coat chicken with flour, followed by eggs and breadcrumbs. Place it in the basket. Spray with a bit of oil and press Start. Cook for 15 minutes.
2. Mix red pepper paste, apple cider vinegar, soy sauce, honey, and ¼ cup water in a saucepan over medium heat and bring the mixture to a boil. Add in the chicken and toss to coat. Garnish with sesame seeds and serve.

167.Delicious Turkey Cutlets

Servings: 4

Cooking Time: 25 Minutes

Ingredients:

- 1 egg
- 1 1/2 lbs turkey cutlets
- 1/2 tsp garlic powder
- 1/2 tsp onion powder
- 1/2 tsp dried parsley
- 1/4 cup parmesan cheese, grated
- 1/2 cup almond flour
- 1/4 tsp pepper
- 1/2 tsp salt

Directions:

1. Fit the oven with the rack in position
2. Add egg in a small bowl and whisk well.
3. In a shallow dish, mix almond flour, parmesan cheese, parsley, onion powder, garlic powder, pepper, and salt.
4. Dip turkey cutlet into the egg and coat with almond flour mixture.
5. Place coated turkey cutlets into the baking pan.
6. Set to bake at 350 F for 30 minutes. After 5 minutes place the baking pan in the preheated oven.
7. Serve and enjoy.

- **Nutrition Info:** Calories 346 Fat 12.6 g Carbohydrates 1.6 g Sugar 0.4 g Protein 53.9 g Cholesterol 174 mg

168.Lush Salisbury Steak With Mushroom Gravy

Servings:2

Cooking Time: 33 Minutes

Ingredients:

- For the Mushroom Gravy:
- ¾ cup sliced button mushrooms
- ¼ cup thinly sliced onions
- ¼ cup unsalted butter, melted
- ½ teaspoon fine sea salt
- ¼ cup beef broth
- For the Steaks:
- ½ pound (227 g) ground beef (85% lean)
- 1 tablespoon dry mustard
- 2 tablespoons tomato paste
- ¼ teaspoon garlic powder
- ½ teaspoon onion powder
- ½ teaspoon fine sea salt
- ¼ teaspoon ground black pepper
- Chopped fresh thyme leaves, for garnish

Directions:

1. Toss the mushrooms and onions with butter in the baking pan to coat well, then sprinkle with salt.
2. Slide the baking pan into Rack Position 1, select Convection Bake, set temperature to 390ºF (199ºC) and set time to 8 minutes.
3. Stir the mixture halfway through the cooking.
4. When cooking is complete, the mushrooms should be tender.
5. Pour the broth in the baking pan and set time to 10 more minutes to make the gravy.
6. Meanwhile, combine all the ingredients for the steaks, except for the thyme leaves, in a

large bowl. Stir to mix well. Shape the mixture into two oval steaks.

7. Arrange the steaks over the gravy and set time to 15 minutes. When cooking is complete, the patties should be browned. Flip the steaks halfway through.
8. Transfer the steaks onto a plate and pour the gravy over. Sprinkle with fresh thyme and serve immediately.

169.Calf's Liver Golden Strips

Servings:4

Cooking Time: 4 To 5 Minutes

Ingredients:

- 1 pound (454 g) sliced calf's liver, cut into about ½-inch-wide strips
- Salt and ground black pepper, to taste
- 2 eggs
- 2 tablespoons milk
- ½ cup whole wheat flour
- 1½ cups panko bread crumbs
- ½ cup plain bread crumbs
- ½ teaspoon salt
- ¼ teaspoon ground black pepper
- Cooking spray

Directions:

1. Sprinkle the liver strips with salt and pepper.
2. Beat together the egg and milk in a bowl. Place wheat flour in a shallow dish. In a second shallow dish, mix panko, plain bread crumbs, ½ teaspoon salt, and ¼ teaspoon pepper.
3. Dip liver strips in flour, egg wash, and then bread crumbs, pressing in coating slightly to make crumbs stick.
4. Spritz the air fryer basket with cooking spray. Place strips in a single layer in the basket.
5. Put the air fryer basket on the baking pan and slide into Rack Position 2, select Air Fry, set the temperature to 400ºF (205ºC) and set the time to 4 minutes.
6. After 2 minutes, remove from the oven. Flip the strips with tongs. Return to the oven and continue cooking.
7. When cooking is complete, the liver strips should be crispy and golden.
8. Serve immediately.

170.One-pot Farfalle Pasta

Servings:x

Cooking Time:x

Ingredients:

- olive oil
- 5 slices bacon, chopped 1 (25-oz) jar marinara sauce with basil
- 2 cups water
- Salt and freshly ground black pepper, to taste
- 2 cups dried farfalle pasta
- 3 cups baby spinach
- 1½ cups fresh Mozzarella cheese, sliced
- Fresh basil leaves
- Grated Parmesan cheese

Directions:

1. Preheat the oven to 375°F.
2. In oven over medium heat, heat the olive oil until hot.
3. Add the bacon crumbles and cook for5 minutes.
4. Add the marinara sauce and water. Bring to a boil. Season with salt and pepper.
5. Add the pasta and spinach, and mix.
6. Tuck a few slices of fresh mozzarella into the mix, and place the rest
7. on top. Cover and bake for 20 minutes, or until the pasta is tender.
8. Sprinkle fresh basil and Parmesan cheese on top, and serve.

171.Spicy Tandoori Chicken Drumsticks

Servings:4

Cooking Time: 14 Minutes

Ingredients:

- 8 (4- to 5-ounce / 113- to 142-g) skinless bone-in chicken drumsticks
- ½ cup plain full-fat or low-fat yogurt
- ¼ cup buttermilk
- 2 teaspoons minced garlic
- 2 teaspoons minced fresh ginger
- 2 teaspoons ground cinnamon
- 2 teaspoons ground coriander
- 2 teaspoons mild paprika
- 1 teaspoon salt
- 1 teaspoon Tabasco hot red pepper sauce

Directions:

1. In a large bowl, stir together all the ingredients except for chicken drumsticks until well combined. Add the chicken drumsticks to the bowl and toss until well coated. Cover in plastic and set in the refrigerator to marinate for 1 hour, tossing once.
2. Arrange the marinated drumsticks in the air fryer basket, leaving enough space between them.
3. Put the air fryer basket on the baking pan and slide into Rack Position 2, select Air Fry, set temperature to 375ºF (190ºC) and set time to 14 minutes.
4. Flip the drumsticks once halfway through to ensure even cooking.
5. When cooking is complete, the internal temperature of the chicken drumsticks should reach 160ºF (71ºC) on a meat thermometer.
6. Transfer the drumsticks to plates. Rest for 5 minutes before serving.

172.Garlic Infused Roast Beef

Servings: 10
Cooking Time: 75 Minutes
Ingredients:

- 3 lb. beef roast, room temperature
- 4 cloves garlic, cut in thin slivers
- Olive oil spray,
- 1 tsp salt
- 1 tsp pepper
- 2 tsp rosemary

Directions:

1. Trim off the fat from the roast. Use a sharp knife to pierce the roast in intervals, ½-inch deep. Insert garlic sliver in holes, pushing into the meat.
2. Lightly spray the beef with oil and season with salt, pepper, and rosemary.
3. Place the baking pan in position 1 of the oven. Set to convection bake on 325°F for 60 minutes.
4. Spray the fryer basket with oil and place roast in it. Once the oven has preheated for 5 minutes, place the basket on the pan. Cook 60 minutes, or until beef reaches desired doneness.
5. Remove from oven and let rest 10 minutes. Slice thinly and serve.

- **Nutrition Info:** Calories 265, Total Fat 13g, Saturated Fat 5g, Total Carbs 1g, Net Carbs 1g, Protein 36g, Sugar 0g, Fiber 0g, Sodium 342mg, Potassium 478mg, Phosphorus 288mg

173.Quail Chili

Servings:x
Cooking Time:x
Ingredients:

- 1 lb. quail (Cut into cubes)
- 2 ½ tsp. ginger-garlic paste
- 1 tsp. red chili sauce
- 2 tbsp. tomato ketchup
- 2 tsp. soya sauce
- 1-2 tbsp. honey
- ¼ tsp. Ajinomoto
- ¼ tsp. salt
- ¼ tsp. red chili powder/black pepper
- A few drops of edible orange food coloring
- 2 tbsp. olive oil
- 1 ½ tsp. ginger garlic paste
- ½ tbsp. red chili sauce
- 1-2 tsp. red chili flakes

Directions:

1. Mix all the ingredients for the marinade and put the quail cubes inside and let it rest overnight.
2. Mix the breadcrumbs, oregano and red chili flakes well and place the marinated Oregano Fingers on this mixture. Cover it with plastic wrap and leave it till right before you serve to cook.
3. Pre heat the oven at 160 degrees Fahrenheit for 5 minutes. Place the Oregano Fingers in the fry basket and close it. Let them cook at the same temperature for another 15 minutes or so. Toss the Oregano Fingers well so that they are cooked uniformly.

174.Ham Club Sandwich

Servings:x
Cooking Time:x

Ingredients:

- 2 slices of white bread
- 1 tbsp. softened butter
- 1 lb. ham (Sliced)
- 1 small capsicum
- For Barbeque Sauce:
- ¼ tbsp. Worcestershire sauce
- ½ tsp. olive oil
- ½ flake garlic crushed
- ¼ tsp. mustard powder
- ¼ cup chopped onion
- ½ tbsp. sugar
- 1 tbsp. tomato ketchup
- ¼ tbsp. red chili sauce
- ½ cup water.
- A pinch of salt and black pepper to taste

Directions:

1. Take the slices of bread and remove the edges. Now cut the slices horizontally. Cook the ingredients for the sauce and wait till it thickens. Now, add the ham slices to the sauce and stir till it obtains the flavors. Roast the capsicum and peel the skin off. Cut the capsicum into slices. Mix the ingredients together and apply it to the bread slices.
2. Pre-heat the oven for 5 minutes at 300 Fahrenheit. Open the basket of the Fryer and place the prepared Classic Sandwiches in it such that no two Classic Sandwiches are touching each other. Now keep the fryer at 250 degrees for around 15 minutes. Turn the Classic Sandwiches in between the cooking process to cook both slices. Serve the Classic Sandwiches with tomato ketchup or mint sauce.

175.Chicken Schnitzel

Servings:4

Cooking Time: 5 Minutes

Ingredients:

- ½ cup all-purpose flour
- 1 teaspoon marjoram
- ½ teaspoon thyme
- 1 teaspoon dried parsley flakes
- ½ teaspoon salt
- 1 egg
- 1 teaspoon lemon juice
- 1 teaspoon water
- 1 cup bread crumbs
- 4 chicken tenders, pounded thin, cut in half lengthwise
- Cooking spray

Directions:

1. Spritz the air fryer basket with cooking spray.
2. Combine the flour, marjoram, thyme, parsley, and salt in a shallow dish. Stir to mix well.
3. Whisk the egg with lemon juice and water in a large bowl. Pour the bread crumbs in a separate shallow dish.
4. Roll the chicken halves in the flour mixture first, then in the egg mixture, and then roll over the bread crumbs to coat well. Shake the excess off.
5. Arrange the chicken halves in the basket and spritz with cooking spray on both sides.
6. Put the air fryer basket on the baking pan and slide into Rack Position 2, select Air Fry, set temperature to 390ºF (199ºC) and set time to 5 minutes.
7. Flip the halves halfway through.
8. When cooking is complete, the chicken halves should be golden brown and crispy.
9. Serve immediately.

176.Garlic Kangaroo

Servings:x

Cooking Time:x

Ingredients:

- 1 lb. boneless kangaroo
- 2 cup dry breadcrumbs
- 2 tsp. oregano
- 2 tsp. red chili flakes
- 2 tsp. garlic paste
- 1 ½ tbsp. ginger-garlic paste
- 4 tbsp. lemon juice
- 2 tsp. salt
- 1 tsp. red chili powder
- 6 tbsp. corn flour
- 4 eggs

Directions:

1. Mix all the ingredients for the marinade and put the kangaroo Oregano Fingers inside and let it rest overnight. Mix the

breadcrumbs, oregano and red chili flakes well and place the marinated Oregano Fingers on this mixture. Cover it with plastic wrap and leave it till right before you serve to cook. Pre heat the oven at 160 degrees Fahrenheit for 5 minutes.

2. Place the Oregano Fingers in the fry basket and close it. Let them cook at the same temperature for another 15 minutes or so. Toss the Oregano Fingers well so that they are cooked uniformly. Drizzle the garlic paste and serve.

177.Pork Wonton Wonderful

Servings: 3
Cooking Time: 25 Minutes
Ingredients:

- 8 wanton wrappers (Leasa brand works great, though any will do)
- 4 ounces of raw minced pork
- 1 medium-sized green apple
- 1 cup of water, for wetting the wanton wrappers
- 1 tablespoon of vegetable oil
- ½ tablespoon of oyster sauce
- 1 tablespoon of soy sauce
- Large pinch of ground white pepper

Directions:

1. Preparing the Ingredients. Cover the basket of the air fryer oven with a lining of tin foil, leaving the edges uncovered to allow air to circulate through the basket. Preheat the air fryer oven to 350 degrees.
2. In a small mixing bowl, combine the oyster sauce, soy sauce, and white pepper, then add in the minced pork and stir thoroughly. Cover and set in the fridge to marinate for at least 15 minutes. Core the apple, and slice into small cubes – smaller than bite-sized chunks.
3. Add the apples to the marinating meat mixture, and combine thoroughly. Spread the wonton wrappers, and fill each with a large spoonful of the filling. Wrap the wontons into triangles, so that the wrappers fully cover the filling, and seal with a drop of the water.
4. Coat each filled and wrapped wonton thoroughly with the vegetable oil, to help ensure a nice crispy fry. Place the wontons on the foil-lined air-fryer rack/basket. Place the Rack on the middle-shelf of the air fryer oven.
5. Air Frying. Set the air fryer oven timer to 25 minutes. Halfway through cooking time, shake the handle of the air fryer rack/basket vigorously to jostle the wontons and ensure even frying. After 25 minutes, when the air fryer oven shuts off, the wontons will be crispy golden-brown on the outside and juicy and delicious on the inside. Serve directly from the Oven rack/basket and enjoy while hot.

178.Basil Cheese Chicken

Servings: 4
Cooking Time: 20 Minutes
Ingredients:

- 4 chicken breasts, cubed
- 1 tbsp garlic powder
- 1 cup mayonnaise
- ½ tsp pepper
- ½ cup soft cheese
- ½ tbsp salt
- Chopped basil for garnish

Directions:

1. In a bowl, mix cheese, mayonnaise, garlic powder, and salt to form a marinade. Cover your chicken with the marinade. Place the marinated chicken in the basket and fit in the baking tray; cook for 15 minutes at 380 F on Air Fry function. Serve garnished with chopped fresh basil.

179.Mustard Chicken Tenders

Servings: 4
Cooking Time: 20 Minutes
Ingredients:

- ½ C. coconut flour
- 1 tbsp. spicy brown mustard
- 2 beaten eggs
- 1 pound of chicken tenders

Directions:

1. Preparing the Ingredients. Season tenders with pepper and salt.

2. Place a thin layer of mustard onto tenders and then dredge in flour and dip in egg.
3. Air Frying. Add to the air fryer oven, set temperature to 390°F, and set time to 20 minutes.

- **Nutrition Info:** CALORIES: 403; FAT: 20G; PROTEIN:22G; SUGAR:4G

180.Bruschetta Chicken

Servings:4
Cooking Time: 10 Minutes
Ingredients:

- Bruschetta Stuffing:
- 1 tomato, diced
- 3 tablespoons balsamic vinegar
- 1 teaspoon Italian seasoning
- 2 tablespoons chopped fresh basil
- 3 garlic cloves, minced
- 2 tablespoons extra-virgin olive oil
- Chicken:
- 4 (4-ounce / 113-g) boneless, skinless chicken breasts, cut 4 slits each
- 1 teaspoon Italian seasoning
- Chicken seasoning or rub, to taste
- Cooking spray

Directions:

1. Spritz the air fryer basket with cooking spray.
2. Combine the ingredients for the bruschetta stuffing in a bowl. Stir to mix well. Set aside.
3. Rub the chicken breasts with Italian seasoning and chicken seasoning on a clean work surface.
4. Arrange the chicken breasts, slits side up, in the basket and spritz with cooking spray.
5. Put the air fryer basket on the baking pan and slide into Rack Position 2, select Air Fry, set temperature to 370ºF (188ºC) and set time to 10 minutes.
6. Flip the breast and fill the slits with the bruschetta stuffing halfway through.
7. When cooking is complete, the chicken should be well browned.
8. Serve immediately.

181.Morning Ham & Cheese Sandwich

Servings: 4
Cooking Time: 15 Minutes
Ingredients:

- 8 slices whole wheat bread
- 4 slices lean pork ham
- 4 slices cheese
- 8 slices tomato

Directions:

1. Lay four slices of bread on a flat surface. Spread the slices with cheese, tomato, turkey, and ham. Cover with the remaining slices to form sandwiches. Add the sandwiches to the cooking basket and cook for 10 minutes at 360 F on Air Fry function. Serve.

182.Poultry Fried Baked Pastry

Servings:x
Cooking Time:x
Ingredients:

- 1 or 2 green chilies that are finely chopped or mashed
- ½ tsp. cumin
- 1 tsp. coarsely crushed coriander
- 1 dry red chili broken into pieces
- A small amount of salt (to taste)
- 2 tbsp. unsalted butter
- 1 ½ cup all-purpose flour
- A pinch of salt to taste
- Water to knead the dough
- 1 lb. mixed minced poultry (squab, chicken, duck, pheasant, turkey)
- ¼ cup boiled peas
- 1 tsp. powdered ginger
- ½ tsp. dried mango powder
- ½ tsp. red chili power.
- 1-2 tbsp. coriander.

Directions:

1. You will first need to make the outer covering. In a large bowl, add the flour, butter and enough water to knead it into dough that is stiff. Transfer this to a container and leave it to rest for five minutes. Place a pan on medium flame and add the oil. Roast the mustard seeds and once roasted, add the coriander seeds and the chopped dry red chilies. Add all the dry ingredients for the filling and mix the ingredients well. Add a little water and

continue to stir the ingredients. Make small balls out of the dough and roll them out.

2. Cut the rolled-out dough into halves and apply a little water on the edges to help you fold the halves into a cone. Add the filling to the cone and close up the samosa. Pre-heat the oven for around 5 to 6 minutes at 300 Fahrenheit. Place all the samosas in the fry basket and close the basket properly. Keep the oven at 200 degrees for another 20 to 25 minutes.
3. Around the halfway point, open the basket and turn the samosas over for uniform cooking. After this, fry at 250 degrees for around 10 minutes in order to give them the desired golden-brown color. Serve hot. Recommended sides are tamarind or mint sauce.

183.Air Fryer Roast Beef

Servings: 6
Cooking Time: 45 Minutes
Ingredients:

- Roast beef
- 1 tbsp. olive oil
- Seasonings of choice

Directions:

1. Preparing the Ingredients. Ensure your air fryer oven is preheated to 160 degrees.
2. Place roast in bowl and toss with olive oil and desired seasonings.
3. Put seasoned roast into the air fryer oven.
4. Air Frying. Set temperature to 160°F, and set time to 30 minutes and cook 30 minutes.
5. Turn roast when the timer sounds and cook another 15 minutes.

- **Nutrition Info:** CALORIES: 267; FAT: 8G; PROTEIN:2G

184.Parmesan Chicken Fingers With Plum Sauce

Servings: 2
Cooking Time: 20 Minutes
Ingredients:

- 2 chicken breasts, cut in strips
- 3 tbsp Parmesan cheese, grated
- ¼ tbsp fresh chives, chopped
- ⅓ cup breadcrumbs
- 1 egg white
- 2 tbsp plum sauce, optional
- ½ tbsp fresh thyme, chopped
- ½ tbsp black pepper
- 1 tbsp water

Directions:

1. Preheat on Air Fry function to 360 F. Mix the chives, Parmesan cheese, thyme, pepper and breadcrumbs. In another bowl, whisk the egg white and mix with the water. Dip the chicken strips into the egg mixture and then in the breadcrumb mixture. Place the strips in the greased basket and fit in the baking tray. Cook for 10 minutes, flipping once. Serve with plum sauce.

185.Smoked Ham With Sweet Glaze

Servings:4
Cooking Time: 30 Minutes
Ingredients:

- 2 pears, chopped
- 1 lb smoked ham
- 1 ½ cups brown sugar
- ¾ tbsp allspice
- 1 tbsp balsamic vinegar
- 1 tsp black pepper

Directions:

1. Preheat oven to 330 F on AirFry function. Place pears, brown sugar, balsamic vinegar, allspices, and pepper in a small pot over medium heat. Stir and bring to a boil then reduce the heat to low. Simmer for 8-10 minutes until the glaze is thickened.
2. Place the ham in a greased baking dish. With a knife, score only the fatty surface of the ham in a diamond pattern. Pour the pear mixture over the ham and cook for 20-25 minutes until golden and glazed. Let sit for a few minutes before slicing and serving.

186.Spice-coated Steaks With Cucumber And Snap Pea Salad

Servings:4
Cooking Time: 15 Minutes
Ingredients:

- 1 (1½-pound / 680-g) boneless top sirloin steak, trimmed and halved crosswise
- 1½ teaspoons chili powder

- 1½ teaspoons ground cumin
- ¾ teaspoon ground coriander
- ⅛ teaspoon cayenne pepper
- ⅛ teaspoon ground cinnamon
- 1¼ teaspoons plus ⅛ teaspoon salt, divided
- ½ teaspoon plus ⅛ teaspoon ground black pepper, divided
- 1 teaspoon plus 1½ tablespoons extra-virgin olive oil, divided
- 3 tablespoons mayonnaise
- 1½ tablespoons white wine vinegar
- 1 tablespoon minced fresh dill
- 1 small garlic clove, minced
- 8 ounces (227 g) sugar snap peas, strings removed and cut in half on bias
- ½ English cucumber, halved lengthwise and sliced thin
- 2 radishes, trimmed, halved and sliced thin
- 2 cups baby arugula

Directions:

1. In a bowl, mix chili powder, cumin, coriander, cayenne pepper, cinnamon, 1¼ teaspoons salt and ½ teaspoon pepper until well combined.
2. Add the steaks to another bowl and pat dry with paper towels. Brush with 1 teaspoon oil and transfer to the bowl of spice mixture. Roll over to coat thoroughly.
3. Arrange the coated steaks in the basket, spaced evenly apart.
4. Put the air fryer basket on the baking pan and slide into Rack Position 2, select Air Fry, set temperature to 400ºF (205ºC) and set time to 15 minutes.
5. Flip the steak halfway through to ensure even cooking.
6. When cooking is complete, an instant-read thermometer inserted in the thickest part of the meat should register at least 145ºF (63ºC).
7. Transfer the steaks to a clean work surface and wrap with aluminum foil. Let stand while preparing salad.
8. Make the salad: In a large bowl, stir together 1½ tablespoons olive oil, mayonnaise, vinegar, dill, garlic, ⅛ teaspoon salt, and ⅛ teaspoon pepper. Add snap peas, cucumber, radishes and arugula. Toss to blend well.
9. Slice the steaks and serve with the salad.

187.Turkey Meatballs

Servings: 4

Cooking Time: 25 Minutes

Ingredients:

- 1 lb ground chicken
- 2 garlic cloves, minced
- 1/2 cup parmesan cheese, grated
- 1/2 cup breadcrumbs
- 1 egg, lightly beaten
- 2 tbsp cilantro, chopped
- 1 tbsp olive oil
- 1/2 tsp red pepper flakes
- 1/4 cup shallots, chopped
- Pepper
- Salt

Directions:

1. Fit the oven with the rack in position
2. Add all ingredients into the large bowl and mix until well combined.
3. Make small balls from the meat mixture and place them into the baking pan.
4. Set to bake at 400 F for 30 minutes. After 5 minutes place the baking pan in the preheated oven.
5. Serve and enjoy.

- **Nutrition Info:** Calories 361 Fat 16.2 g Carbohydrates 12.6 g Sugar 1 g Protein 40 g Cholesterol 150 mg

188.Pork Tandoor

Servings:x

Cooking Time:x

Ingredients:

- 2 cup fresh green coriander
- ½ cup mint leaves
- 4 tsp. fennel
- 2 tbsp. ginger-garlic paste
- 1 small onion
- 2 cups sliced pork belly
- 1 big capsicum (Cut this capsicum into big cubes)
- 1 onion (Cut it into quarters. Now separate the layers carefully.)
- 5 tbsp. gram flour

- A pinch of salt to taste
- 6-7 flakes garlic (optional)
- Salt to taste
- 3 tbsp. lemon juice

Directions:

1. You will first need to make the sauce. Add the ingredients to a blender and make a thick paste. Slit the pieces of pork and stuff half the paste into the cavity obtained. Take the remaining paste and add it to the gram flour and salt. Toss the pieces of Pork in this mixture and set aside. Apply a little bit of the mixture on the capsicum and onion.
2. Place these on a stick along with the pork pieces. Pre heat the oven at 290 Fahrenheit for around 5 minutes. Open the basket. Arrange the satay sticks properly.
3. Close the basket. Keep the sticks with the pork at 180 degrees for around half an hour while the sticks with the vegetables are to be kept at the same temperature for only 7 minutes. Turn the sticks in between so that one side does not get burnt and also to provide a uniform cook.

189.Herb Pork Tenderloin

Servings: 4
Cooking Time: 35 Minutes
Ingredients:

- 1 lb pork tenderloin
- 1/2 tbsp dried rosemary
- 1/2 tsp dried thyme
- 1 tbsp olive oil
- Pepper
- Salt

Directions:

1. Fit the oven with the rack in position
2. Mix rosemary, thyme, oil, pepper, and salt and rub over pork tenderloin.
3. Place pork tenderloin in baking pan.
4. Set to bake at 400 F for 40 minutes. After 5 minutes place the baking pan in the preheated oven.
5. Slice and serve.

- **Nutrition Info:** Calories 194 Fat 7.6 g Carbohydrates 0.4 g Sugar 0 g Protein 29.7 g Cholesterol 83 mg

190.Green Chili Chicken Noodle Casserole

Servings: 6
Cooking Time: 30 Minutes
Ingredients:

- 3 cups cooked chicken, shredded
- 4 oz can green chilies
- 1/3 cup parmesan cheese, shredded
- 3 cups cheddar cheese, shredded
- 1 1/3 cups milk
- 10.5 oz cream of chicken soup
- 1 tsp chili powder
- 1 onion, diced
- 1/3 cup bell pepper, diced
- 3 tbsp butter
- 3 cups shell noodles, uncooked
- 1/2 tsp salt

Directions:

1. Fit the oven with the rack in position
2. Cook noodles according to the packet instructions and drain well.
3. Melt butter in a pan over medium heat.
4. Add bell pepper and onion and sauté for 5 minutes. Stir in chili powder and salt.
5. In a large bowl, mix chicken soup, parmesan cheese, 2 cups cheddar cheese, milk, and sautéed onion bell pepper. Stir in green chilies, noodles, and chicken.
6. Pour mixture into the greased 9*13-inch baking dish and top with remaining cheese.
7. Set to bake at 375 F for 35 minutes. After 5 minutes place the baking dish in the preheated oven.
8. Serve and enjoy.

- **Nutrition Info:** Calories 560 Fat 32.6 g Carbohydrates 23.9 g Sugar 5 g Protein 42.2 g Cholesterol 156 mg

191.Country Fried Steak

Servings: 2
Cooking Time: 12 Minutes
Ingredients:

- 1 tsp. pepper
- 2 C. almond milk
- 2 tbsp. almond flour
- 6 ounces ground sausage meat
- 1 tsp. pepper
- 1 tsp. salt

- 1 tsp. garlic powder
- 1 tsp. onion powder
- 1 C. panko breadcrumbs
- 1 C. almond flour
- 3 beaten eggs
- 6 ounces sirloin steak, pounded till thin

Directions:

1. Preparing the Ingredients. Season panko breadcrumbs with spices.
2. Dredge steak in flour, then egg, and then seasoned panko mixture.
3. Place into air fryer rack/basket.
4. Air Frying. Set temperature to 370°F, and set time to 12 minutes.
5. To make sausage gravy, cook sausage and drain off fat, but reserve 2 tablespoons.
6. Add flour to sausage and mix until incorporated. Gradually mix in milk over medium to high heat till it becomes thick.
7. Season mixture with pepper and cook 3 minutes longer.
8. Serve steak topped with gravy and enjoy!

- **Nutrition Info:** CALORIES: 395; FAT: 11G; PROTEIN:39G; SUGAR:5G

192.Asian Meatballs

Servings: 4

Cooking Time: 15 Minutes

Ingredients:

- 1 lb ground pork
- 1/2 lime juice
- 2 tsp curry paste
- 1 tbsp Worcestershire sauce
- 1 tbsp soy sauce
- 1 tsp garlic puree
- 1 tsp coriander
- 1 tsp Chinese spice
- 1 tsp mixed spice
- 1 onion, chopped
- Pepper
- Salt

Directions:

1. Fit the oven with the rack in position 2.
2. Line the air fryer basket with parchment paper.
3. Add all ingredients into a large bowl and mix until well combined.
4. Make small balls from meat mixture and place in the air fryer basket then place an air fryer basket in the baking pan.
5. Place a baking pan on the oven rack. Set to air fry at 350 F for 15 minutes.
6. Serve and enjoy.

- **Nutrition Info:** Calories 199 Fat 5.7 g Carbohydrates 4.8 g Sugar 2.1 g Protein 30.4 g Cholesterol 83 mg

193.Crispy Mongolian Beef

Servings: 6

Cooking Time: 10 Minutes

Ingredients:

- Olive oil
- ½ C. almond flour
- 2 pounds beef tenderloin or beef chuck, sliced into strips
- Sauce:
- ½ C. chopped green onion
- 1 tsp. red chili flakes
- 1 tsp. almond flour
- ½ C. brown sugar
- 1 tsp. hoisin sauce
- ½ C. water
- ½ C. rice vinegar
- ½ C. low-sodium soy sauce
- 1 tbsp. chopped garlic
- 1 tbsp. finely chopped ginger
- 2 tbsp. olive oil

Directions:

1. Preparing the Ingredients. Toss strips of beef in almond flour, ensuring they are coated well. Add to the air fryer oven.
2. Air Frying. Set temperature to 300°F, and set time to 10 minutes, and cook 10 minutes at 300 degrees.
3. Meanwhile, add all sauce ingredients to the pan and bring to a boil. Mix well.
4. Add beef strips to the sauce and cook 2 minutes.
5. Serve over cauliflower rice!

- **Nutrition Info:** CALORIES: 290; FAT: 14G; PROTEIN:22G; SUGAR:1G

194.Chicken Marinade Cutlet

Servings:x

Cooking Time:x

Ingredients:

- 2 cups sliced chicken
- 4 tsp. fennel
- 2 tbsp. ginger-garlic paste
- 1 small onion
- 6-7 flakes garlic (optional)
- Salt to taste
- 1 big capsicum (Cut this capsicum into big cubes)
- 1 onion (Cut it into quarters. Now separate the layers carefully.)
- 5 tbsp. gram flour
- A pinch of salt to taste
- 2 cup fresh green coriander
- ½ cup mint leaves
- 3 tbsp. lemon juice

Directions:

1. You will first need to make the sauce. Add the ingredients to a blender and make a thick paste. Slit the pieces of chicken and stuff half the paste into the cavity obtained.
2. Take the remaining paste and add it to the gram flour and salt. Toss the pieces of chicken in this mixture and set aside.
3. Apply a little bit of the mixture on the capsicum and onion. Place these on a stick along with the chicken pieces.
4. Pre heat the oven at 290 Fahrenheit for around 5 minutes. Open the basket. Arrange the satay sticks properly. Close the basket. Keep the sticks with the chicken at 180 degrees for around half an hour while the sticks with the vegetables are to be kept at the same temperature for only 7 minutes. Turn the sticks in between so that one side does not get burnt and also to provide a uniform cook.

195.Cracker Apple Chicken

Servings: 2

Cooking Time: 45 Minutes

Ingredients:

- 2 chicken breasts, skinless and boneless
- 1 apple, sliced
- 12 Ritz cracker, crushed
- 10 oz can condensed cheddar cheese soup
- Pepper
- Salt

Directions:

1. Fit the oven with the rack in position
2. Season chicken with pepper and salt and place into the baking dish.
3. Arrange sliced apple on top of chicken.
4. Sprinkle crushed crackers on top.
5. Set to bake at 350 F for 50 minutes. After 5 minutes place the baking dish in the preheated oven.
6. Pour cheddar cheese soup on top and serve.

- **Nutrition Info:** Calories 924 Fat 38.2 g Carbohydrates 87 g Sugar 21.4 g Protein 51.8 g Cholesterol 136 mg

FISH & SEAFOOD RECIPES

196.Lobster Grandma's Easy To Cook Wontons

Servings:x
Cooking Time:x
Ingredients:

- 1 ½ cup all-purpose flour
- ½ tsp. salt
- 5 tbsp. water
- For filling:
- 2 cups minced lobster
- 2 tbsp. oil
- 2 tsp. ginger-garlic paste
- 2 tsp. soya sauce
- 2 tsp. vinegar

Directions:

1. Squeeze the dough and cover it with plastic wrap and set aside. Next, cook the ingredients for the filling and try to ensure that the lobster is covered well with the sauce.
2. Roll the dough and place the filling in the center. Now, wrap the dough to cover the filling and pinch the edges together.
3. Pre heat the oven at 200° F for 5 minutes. Place the wontons in the fry basket and close it. Let them cook at the same temperature for another 20 minutes. Recommended sides are chili sauce or ketchup.

197.Seafood Pizza

Servings:x
Cooking Time:x
Ingredients:

- One pizza base
- Grated pizza cheese (mozzarella cheese preferably) for topping
- Some pizza topping sauce
- Use cooking oil for brushing and topping purposes
- ingredients for topping:
- 2 onions chopped
- 2 cups mixed seafood
- 2 capsicums chopped
- 2 tomatoes that have been deseeded and chopped
- 1 tbsp. (optional) mushrooms/corns
- 2 tsp. pizza seasoning
- Some cottage cheese that has been cut into small cubes (optional)

Directions:

1. Put the pizza base in a pre-heated oven for around 5 minutes. (Pre heated to 340 Fahrenheit). Take out the base. Pour some pizza sauce on top of the base at the center. Using a spoon spread the sauce over the base making sure that you leave some gap around the circumference. Grate some mozzarella cheese and sprinkle it over the sauce layer. Take all the vegetables and the seafood and mix them in a bowl. Add some oil and seasoning.
2. Also add some salt and pepper according to taste. Mix them properly. Put this topping over the layer of cheese on the pizza. Now sprinkle some more grated cheese and pizza seasoning on top of this layer. Pre heat the oven at 250 Fahrenheit for around 5 minutes.
3. Open the fry basket and place the pizza inside. Close the basket and keep the fryer at 170 degrees for another 10 minutes. If you feel that it is undercooked you may put it at the same temperature for another 2 minutes or so.

198.Cheese Carp Fries

Servings:x
Cooking Time:x
Ingredients:

- 1 lb. carp Oregano Fingers
- ingredients for the marinade:
- 1 tbsp. olive oil
- 1 tsp. mixed herbs
- ½ tsp. red chili flakes
- A pinch of salt to taste
- 1 tbsp. lemon juice
- For the garnish:
- 1 cup melted cheddar cheese

Directions:

1. Take all the ingredients mentioned under the heading "For the marinade" and mix them well. Cook the carp Oregano Fingers and soak them in the marinade.
2. Pre heat the oven for around 5 minutes at 300 Fahrenheit. Take out the basket of the fryer and place the carp in them. Close the basket. Now keep the fryer at 220 Fahrenheit for 20 or 25 minutes.
3. In between the process, toss the fries twice or thrice so that they get cooked properly. Towards the end of the cooking process (the last 2 minutes or so), sprinkle the melted cheddar cheese over the fries and serve hot.

199.Baked Buttery Shrimp

Servings: 4
Cooking Time: 15 Minutes
Ingredients:

- 1 lb shrimp, peel & deveined
- 2 tsp garlic powder
- 2 tsp dry mustard
- 2 tsp cumin
- 2 tsp paprika
- 2 tsp black pepper
- 4 tsp cayenne pepper
- 1/2 cup butter, melted
- 2 tsp onion powder
- 1 tsp dried oregano
- 1 tsp dried thyme
- 3 tsp salt

Directions:

1. Fit the oven with the rack in position
2. Add shrimp, butter, and remaining ingredients into the mixing bowl and toss well.
3. Transfer shrimp mixture into the baking pan.
4. Set to bake at 400 F for 20 minutes. After 5 minutes place the baking pan in the preheated oven.
5. Serve and enjoy.

- **Nutrition Info:** Calories 372 Fat 26.2 g Carbohydrates 7.5 g Sugar 1.3 g Protein 27.6 g Cholesterol 300 mg

200.Crispy Salmon With Lemon-butter Sauce

Servings:x
Cooking Time:x
Ingredients:

- 4 (4-6-oz) salmon fillets, patted dry
- Salt and pepper, to taste
- 2 Tbsp olive oil
- 1 large garlic clove, minced
- 1/3 cup dry white wine
- 2 Tbsp fresh lemon juice
- 1 lemon zested
- 3 Tbsp unsalted butter, diced
- 2 Tbsp chopped fresh dill

Directions:

1. Place oven over medium heat.
2. Sprinkle salt and pepper on salmon fillets and add 1 Tbsp oil to the pan.
3. Add salmon flesh side down and cook 3-4 minutes. Flip the salmon and cook an additional 3 minutes on skin side. Transfer to a plate.
4. Wipe out oven and add remaining Tbsp olive oil over medium heat.
5. Add garlic and saute for 1 minute.
6. Pour in white wine and lemon juice. Stir for one minute.
7. Add lemon zest and continue stirring until slightly reduced.
8. Reduce heat to low and add cubed butter, stirring after each addition.
9. Sprinkle in fresh dill and stir all together.
10. Season with salt and pepper and pour sauce over salmon fillets.

201.Lemon-honey Snapper With Fruit

Servings:4
Cooking Time: 12 Minutes
Ingredients:

- 4 (4-ounce / 113-g) red snapper fillets
- 2 teaspoons olive oil
- 3 plums, halved and pitted
- 3 nectarines, halved and pitted
- 1 cup red grapes
- 1 tablespoon freshly squeezed lemon juice
- 1 tablespoon honey
- ½ teaspoon dried thyme

Directions:

1. Arrange the red snapper fillets in the air fryer basket and drizzle the olive oil over the top.
2. Put the air fryer basket on the baking pan and slide into Rack Position 2, select Air Fry, set temperature to 390ºF (199ºC), and set time to 12 minutes.
3. After 4 minutes, remove from the oven. Top the fillets with the plums and nectarines. Scatter the red grapes all over the fillets. Drizzle with the lemon juice and honey and sprinkle the thyme on top. Return the pan to the oven and continue cooking for 8 minutes, or until the fish is flaky.
4. When cooking is complete, remove from the oven and serve warm.

202.Basil Tomato Salmon

Servings: 2
Cooking Time: 20 Minutes
Ingredients:

- 2 salmon fillets
- 1 tomato, sliced
- 1 tbsp dried basil
- 2 tbsp parmesan cheese, grated
- 1 tbsp olive oil

Directions:

1. Fit the oven with the rack in position
2. Place salmon fillets in a baking dish.
3. Sprinkle basil on top of salmon fillets.
4. Arrange tomato slices on top of salmon fillets. Drizzle with oil and top with cheese.
5. Set to bake at 375 F for 25 minutes. After 5 minutes place the baking dish in the preheated oven.
6. Serve and enjoy.

- **Nutrition Info:** Calories 324 Fat 19.6 g Carbohydrates 1.5 g Sugar 0.8 g Protein 37.1 g Cholesterol 83 mg

203.Flavorful Herb Salmon

Servings: 4
Cooking Time: 15 Minutes
Ingredients:

- 1 lb salmon fillets
- 1/2 tbsp dried rosemary
- 1 tbsp olive oil
- 1/4 tsp dried basil
- 1 tbsp dried chives
- 1/4 tsp dried thyme
- Pepper
- Salt

Directions:

1. Fit the oven with the rack in position 2.
2. Place salmon skin side down in air fryer basket then place an air fryer basket in baking pan.
3. Mix olive oil, thyme, basil, chives, and rosemary in a small bowl.
4. Brush salmon with oil mixture.
5. Place a baking pan on the oven rack. Set to air fry at 400 F for 15 minutes.
6. Serve and enjoy.

- **Nutrition Info:** Calories 182 Fat 10.6 g Carbohydrates 0.4 g Sugar 0 g Protein 22.1 g Cholesterol 50 mg

204.Spicy Baked Shrimp

Servings: 4
Cooking Time: 8 Minutes
Ingredients:

- 2 lbs shrimp, peeled & deveined
- 1/4 tsp cayenne pepper
- 1 tsp garlic powder
- 2 tbsp chili powder
- 2 tbsp olive oil
- 1 tsp kosher salt

Directions:

1. Fit the oven with the rack in position
2. Toss shrimp with remaining ingredients.
3. Transfer shrimp into the baking pan.
4. Set to bake at 400 F for 13 minutes. After 5 minutes place the baking pan in the preheated oven.
5. Serve and enjoy.

- **Nutrition Info:** Calories 344 Fat 11.5 g Carbohydrates 6.1 g Sugar 0.5 g Protein 52.3 g Cholesterol 478 mg

205.Baked Garlic Tilapia

Servings: 4
Cooking Time: 15 Minutes
Ingredients:

- 1 lb tilapia fillets
- 2 tbsp garlic, minced

- 2 tbsp olive oil
- 2 tbsp dried parsley
- Pepper
- Salt

Directions:

1. Fit the oven with the rack in position
2. Place fish fillets in a baking dish. Drizzle with oil and season with pepper and salt.
3. Sprinkle garlic and parsley over fish fillets.
4. Set to bake at 400 F for 20 minutes. After 5 minutes place the baking dish in the preheated oven.
5. Serve and enjoy.

- **Nutrition Info:** Calories 160 Fat 8.1 g Carbohydrates 1.5 g Sugar 0.1 g Protein 21.4 g Cholesterol 55 mg

206.Baked Tilapia With Garlic Aioli

Servings:4

Cooking Time: 15 Minutes

Ingredients:

- Tilapia:
- 4 tilapia fillets
- 1 tablespoon extra-virgin olive oil
- 1 teaspoon garlic powder
- 1 teaspoon paprika
- 1 teaspoon dried basil
- A pinch of lemon-pepper seasoning
- Garlic Aioli:
- 2 garlic cloves, minced
- 1 tablespoon mayonnaise
- Juice of ½ lemon
- 1 teaspoon extra-virgin olive oil
- Salt and pepper, to taste

Directions:

1. On a clean work surface, brush both sides of each fillet with the olive oil. Sprinkle with the garlic powder, paprika, basil, and lemon-pepper seasoning. Place the fillets in the baking pan.
2. Slide the baking pan into Rack Position 1, select Convection Bake, set temperature to 400ºF (205ºC), and set time to 15 minutes.
3. Flip the fillets halfway through.
4. Meanwhile, make the garlic aioli: Whisk together the garlic, mayo, lemon juice, olive oil, salt, and pepper in a small bowl until smooth.
5. When cooking is complete, the fish should flake apart with a fork and no longer translucent in the center. Remove the fish from the oven and serve with the garlic aioli on the side.

207.Flavorful Baked Halibut

Servings: 4

Cooking Time: 12 Minutes

Ingredients:

- 1 lb halibut fillets
- 1/4 tsp garlic powder
- 1/4 tsp paprika
- 1/4 tsp smoked paprika
- 1/4 tsp pepper
- 1/4 cup olive oil
- 1 lemon juice
- 1/2 tsp salt

Directions:

1. Fit the oven with the rack in position
2. Place fish fillets into the baking dish.
3. In a small bowl, mix lemon juice, oil, paprika, smoked paprika, garlic powder, and salt.
4. Brush lemon juice mixture over fish fillets.
5. Set to bake at 425 F for 17 minutes. After 5 minutes place the baking dish in the preheated oven.
6. Serve and enjoy.

- **Nutrition Info:** Calories 236 Fat 15.3 g Carbohydrates 0.4 g Sugar 0.1 g Protein 24 g Cholesterol 36 mg

208.Sticky Hoisin Tuna

Servings:4

Cooking Time: 5 Minutes

Ingredients:

- ½ cup hoisin sauce
- 2 tablespoons rice wine vinegar
- 2 teaspoons sesame oil
- 2 teaspoons dried lemongrass
- 1 teaspoon garlic powder
- ¼ teaspoon red pepper flakes
- ½ small onion, quartered and thinly sliced
- 8 ounces (227 g) fresh tuna, cut into 1-inch cubes
- Cooking spray
- 3 cups cooked jasmine rice

Directions:

1. In a small bowl, whisk together the hoisin sauce, vinegar, sesame oil, lemongrass, garlic powder, and red pepper flakes.
2. Add the sliced onion and tuna cubes and gently toss until the fish is evenly coated.
3. Arrange the coated tuna cubes in the air fryer basket in a single layer.
4. Put the air fryer basket on the baking pan and slide into Rack Position 2, select Air Fry, set temperature to 390ºF (199ºC), and set time to 5 minutes.
5. Flip the fish halfway through the cooking time.
6. When cooking is complete, the fish should begin to flake. Continue cooking for 1 minute, if necessary. Remove from the oven and serve over hot jasmine rice.

209.Garlic-butter Shrimp With Vegetables

Servings:4
Cooking Time: 15 Minutes
Ingredients:

- 1 pound (454 g) small red potatoes, halved
- 2 ears corn, shucked and cut into rounds, 1 to 1½ inches thick
- 2 tablespoons Old Bay or similar seasoning
- ½ cup unsalted butter, melted
- 1 (12- to 13-ounce / 340- to 369-g) package kielbasa or other smoked sausages
- 3 garlic cloves, minced
- 1 pound (454 g) medium shrimp, peeled and deveined

Directions:

1. Place the potatoes and corn in a large bowl.
2. Stir together the butter and Old Bay seasoning in a small bowl. Drizzle half the butter mixture over the potatoes and corn, tossing to coat. Spread out the vegetables in the baking pan.
3. Slide the baking pan into Rack Position 2, select Roast, set temperature to 350ºF (180ºC), and set time to 15 minutes.
4. Meanwhile, cut the sausages into 2-inch lengths, then cut each piece in half lengthwise. Put the sausages and shrimp in a medium bowl and set aside.
5. Add the garlic to the bowl of remaining butter mixture and stir well.
6. After 10 minutes, remove the pan and pour the vegetables into the large bowl. Drizzle with the garlic butter and toss until well coated. Arrange the vegetables, sausages, and shrimp in the pan.
7. Return to the oven and continue cooking. After 5 minutes, check the shrimp for doneness. The shrimp should be pink and opaque. If they are not quite cooked through, roast for an additional 1 minute.
8. When done, remove from the oven and serve on a plate.

210.Roasted Scallops With Snow Peas

Servings:4
Cooking Time: 8 Minutes
Ingredients:

- 1 pound (454 g) sea scallops
- 3 tablespoons hoisin sauce
- ½ cup toasted sesame seeds
- 6 ounces (170 g) snow peas, trimmed
- 3 teaspoons vegetable oil, divided
- 1 teaspoon soy sauce
- 1 teaspoon sesame oil
- 1 cup roasted mushrooms

Directions:

1. Brush the scallops with the hoisin sauce. Put the sesame seeds in a shallow dish. Roll the scallops in the sesame seeds until evenly coated.
2. Combine the snow peas with 1 teaspoon of vegetable oil, the sesame oil, and soy sauce in a medium bowl and toss to coat.
3. Grease the baking pan with the remaining 2 teaspoons of vegetable oil. Put the scallops in the middle of the pan and arrange the snow peas around the scallops in a single layer.
4. Slide the baking pan into Rack Position 2, select Roast, set temperature to 375ºF (190ºC), and set time to 8 minutes.
5. After 5 minutes, remove the pan and flip the scallops. Fold in the mushrooms and stir well. Return the pan to the oven and continue cooking.
6. When done, remove from the oven and cool for 5 minutes. Serve warm.

211.Salmon Beans & Mushrooms

Servings: 6
Cooking Time: 25 Minutes
Ingredients:

- 4 salmon fillets
- 2 tbsp fresh parsley, minced
- 1/4 cup fresh lemon juice
- 1 tsp garlic, minced
- 1 tbsp olive oil
- 1/2 lb mushrooms, sliced
- 1/2 lb green beans, trimmed
- 1/2 cup parmesan cheese, grated
- Pepper
- Salt

Directions:

1. Fit the oven with the rack in position
2. Heat oil in a small saucepan over medium-high heat.
3. Add garlic and sauté for 30 seconds.
4. Remove from heat and stir in lemon juice, parsley, pepper, and salt.
5. Arrange fish fillets, mushrooms, and green beans in baking pan and drizzle with oil mixture.
6. Sprinkle with grated parmesan cheese.
7. Set to bake at 400 F for 30 minutes. After 5 minutes place the baking pan in the preheated oven.
8. Serve and enjoy.

- **Nutrition Info:** Calories 225 Fat 11.5 g Carbohydrates 4.7 g Sugar 1.4 g Protein 27.5 g Cholesterol 58 mg

212.Fish And Chips

Servings: 4
Cooking Time: 20 Minutes
Ingredients:

- 4 (4-ounce) fish fillets
- Pinch salt
- Freshly ground black pepper
- ½ teaspoon dried thyme
- 1 egg white
- ¾ cup crushed potato chips
- 2 tablespoons olive oil, divided
- 1 russet potatoes, peeled and cut into strips

Directions:

1. Preparing the Ingredients. Pat the fish fillets dry and sprinkle with salt, pepper, and thyme. Set aside.
2. In a shallow bowl, beat the egg white until foamy. In another bowl, combine the potato chips and 1 tablespoon of olive oil and mix until combined.
3. Dip the fish fillets into the egg white, then into the crushed potato chip mixture to coat.
4. Toss the fresh potato strips with the remaining 1 tablespoon olive oil.
5. Air Frying. Use your separator to divide the Oven rack/basket in half, then fry the chips and fish. The chips will take about 20 minutes; the fish will take about 10 to 12 minutes to cook.

- **Nutrition Info:** CALORIES: 374; FAT:16G; PROTEIN:30G; FIBER:4G

213.Tasty Tuna Loaf

Servings: 6
Cooking Time: 40 Minutes
Ingredients:

- Nonstick cooking spray
- 12 oz. can chunk white tuna in water, drain & flake
- ¾ cup bread crumbs
- 1 onion, chopped fine
- 2 eggs, beaten
- ¼ cup milk
- ½ tsp fresh lemon juice
- ½ tsp dill
- 1 tbsp. fresh parsley, chopped
- ½ tsp salt
- ½ tsp pepper

Directions:

1. Place rack in position 1 of the oven. Spray a 9-inch loaf pan with cooking spray.
2. In a large bowl, combine all ingredients until thoroughly mixed. Spread evenly in prepared pan.
3. Set oven to bake on 350°F for 45 minutes. After 5 minutes, place the pan in the oven and cook 40 minutes, or until top is golden brown. Slice and serve.

- **Nutrition Info:** Calories 169, Total Fat 5g, Saturated Fat 1g, Total Carbs 13g, Net Carbs 12g, Protein 18g, Sugar 3g, Fiber 1g, Sodium

540mg, Potassium 247mg, Phosphorus 202mg

214.Fish Cakes With Mango Relish

Servings: 4

Cooking Time: 10 Minutes

Ingredients:

- 1 lb White Fish Fillets
- 3 Tbsps Ground Coconut
- 1 Ripened Mango
- ½ Tsps Chili Paste
- Tbsps Fresh Parsley
- 1 Green Onion
- 1 Lime
- 1 Tsp Salt
- 1 Egg

Directions:

1. Preparing the Ingredients. To make the relish, peel and dice the mango into cubes. Combine with a half teaspoon of chili paste, a tablespoon of parsley, and the zest and juice of half a lime.
2. In a food processor, pulse the fish until it forms a smooth texture. Place into a bowl and add the salt, egg, chopped green onion, parsley, two tablespoons of the coconut, and the remainder of the chili paste and lime zest and juice. Combine well
3. Portion the mixture into 10 equal balls and flatten them into small patties. Pour the reserved tablespoon of coconut onto a dish and roll the patties over to coat.
4. Preheat the Air fryer oven to 390 degrees
5. Air Frying. Place the fish cakes into the air fryer oven and cook for 8 minutes. They should be crisp and lightly browned when ready
6. Serve hot with mango relish

215.Mustard-crusted Sole Fillets

Servings:4

Cooking Time: 10 Minutes

Ingredients:

- 5 teaspoons low-sodium yellow mustard
- 1 tablespoon freshly squeezed lemon juice
- 4 (3.5-ounce / 99-g) sole fillets
- 2 teaspoons olive oil
- ½ teaspoon dried marjoram
- ½ teaspoon dried thyme
- ⅛ teaspoon freshly ground black pepper
- 1 slice low-sodium whole-wheat bread, crumbled

Directions:

1. Whisk together the mustard and lemon juice in a small bowl until thoroughly mixed and smooth. Spread the mixture evenly over the sole fillets, then transfer the fillets to the baking pan.
2. In a separate bowl, combine the olive oil, marjoram, thyme, black pepper, and bread crumbs and stir to mix well. Gently but firmly press the mixture onto the top of fillets, coating them completely.
3. Slide the baking pan into Rack Position 1, select Convection Bake, set temperature to 320ºF (160ºC), and set time to 10 minutes.
4. When cooking is complete, the fish should reach an internal temperature of 145ºF (63ºC) on a meat thermometer. Remove from the oven and serve on a plate.

216.Soy And Ginger Shrimp

Servings: 4

Cooking Time: 10 Minutes

Ingredients:

- 2 tablespoons olive oil
- 2 tablespoons scallions, finely chopped
- 2 cloves garlic, chopped
- 1 teaspoon fresh ginger, grated
- 1 tablespoon dry white wine
- 1 tablespoon balsamic vinegar
- 1/4 cup soy sauce
- 1 tablespoon sugar
- 1 pound shrimp
- Salt and ground black pepper, to taste

Directions:

1. Preparing the Ingredients. To make the marinade, warm the oil in a saucepan; cook all ingredients, except the shrimp, salt, and black pepper. Now, let it cool.
2. Marinate the shrimp, covered, at least an hour, in the refrigerator.
3. Air Frying. After that, bake the shrimp at 350 degrees F for 8 to 10 minutes (depending on the size), turning once or

twice. Season prepared shrimp with salt and black pepper and serve right away.

217.Spicy Orange Shrimp

Servings:4
Cooking Time: 12 Minutes
Ingredients:

- $^{1}/_{3}$ cup orange juice
- 3 teaspoons minced garlic
- 1 teaspoon Old Bay seasoning
- ¼ to ½ teaspoon cayenne pepper
- 1 pound (454 g) medium shrimp, thawed, deveined, peeled, with tails off, and patted dry
- Cooking spray

Directions:

1. Stir together the orange juice, garlic, Old Bay seasoning, and cayenne pepper in a medium bowl. Add the shrimp to the bowl and toss to coat well.
2. Cover the bowl with plastic wrap and marinate in the refrigerator for 30 minutes.
3. Spritz the air fryer basket with cooking spray. Place the shrimp in the pan and spray with cooking spray.
4. Put the air fryer basket on the baking pan and slide into Rack Position 2, select Air Fry, set temperature to 400ºF (205ºC), and set time to 12 minutes.
5. Flip the shrimp halfway through the cooking time.
6. When cooked, the shrimp should be opaque and crisp. Remove from the oven and serve hot.

218.Homemade Fish Sticks

Servings: 8 Fish Sticks
Cooking Time: 8 Minutes
Ingredients:

- 8 ounces (227 g) fish fillets (pollock or cod), cut into ½×3-inch strips
- Salt, to taste (optional)
- ½ cup plain bread crumbs
- Cooking spray

Directions:

1. Season the fish strips with salt to taste, if desired.
2. Place the bread crumbs on a plate. Roll the fish strips in the bread crumbs to coat. Spritz the fish strips with cooking spray.
3. Arrange the fish strips in the air fryer basket in a single layer.
4. Put the air fryer basket on the baking pan and slide into Rack Position 2, select Air Fry, set temperature to 390ºF (199ºC), and set time to 8 minutes.
5. When cooking is complete, they should be golden brown. Remove from the oven and cool for 5 minutes before serving.

219.Lemon Tilapia

Servings:4
Cooking Time: 12 Minutes
Ingredients:

- 1 tablespoon olive oil
- 1 tablespoon lemon juice
- 1 teaspoon minced garlic
- ½ teaspoon chili powder
- 4 tilapia fillets

Directions:

1. Line the baking pan with parchment paper.
2. In a shallow bowl, stir together the olive oil, lemon juice, garlic, and chili powder to make a marinade. Put the tilapia fillets in the bowl, turning to coat evenly.
3. Place the fillets in the baking pan in a single layer.
4. Put the air fryer basket on the baking pan and slide into Rack Position 2, select Air Fry, set temperature to 375ºF (190ºC), and set time to 12 minutes.
5. When cooked, the fish will flake apart with a fork. Remove from the oven to a plate and serve hot.

220.Air Fried Haddock Filets

Servings: 8
Cooking Time: 20 Minutes
Ingredients:

- Nonstick cooking spray
- 2 egg whites
- ½ tsp dill
- ½ tsp pepper
- 1 cup cornflakes, crushed
- 2 lbs. haddock fillets, cut in 8 pieces

Directions:

1. Place baking pan in position 2 of the oven. Lightly spray fryer basket with cooking spray.
2. In a shallow bowl, whisk together egg whites, dill, and pepper.
3. Place crushed cornflakes in a separate shallow dish.
4. Dip fish in egg mixture, then cornflakes, coating completely. Place in fryer basket.
5. Place basket on the baking pan and set oven to air fryer on 400°F. Cook 18-20 minutes, turning over halfway through, until fish flakes easily with a fork. Serve.

- **Nutrition Info:** Calories 193, Total Fat 1g, Saturated Fat 0g, Total Carbs 7g, Net Carbs 7g, Protein 39g, Sugar 1g, Fiber 0g, Sodium 568mg, Potassium 692mg, Phosphorus 524mg

221.Baked Tilapia

Servings: 4

Cooking Time: 10 Minutes

Ingredients:

- 1 1/4 lbs tilapia fillets
- 2 tsp onion powder
- 2 tbsp olive oil
- 1/2 tsp garlic powder
- 1/2 tsp dried thyme
- 1/2 tsp oregano
- 1/2 tsp chili powder
- 2 tbsp sweet paprika
- 1 tsp pepper
- 1/2 tsp salt

Directions:

1. Fit the oven with the rack in position
2. Brush fish fillets with oil and place in baking dish.
3. Mix together spices and sprinkle over the fish fillets.
4. Set to bake at 425 F for 15 minutes. After 5 minutes place the baking dish in the preheated oven.
5. Serve and enjoy.

- **Nutrition Info:** Calories 195 Fat 8.9 g Carbohydrates 3.9 g Sugar 0.9 g Protein 27.2 g Cholesterol 69 mg

222.Oyster Club Sandwich

Servings:x

Cooking Time:x

Ingredients:

- 2 slices of white bread
- 1 tbsp. softened butter
- ½ lb. shelled oyster
- 1 small capsicum
- For Barbeque Sauce:
- ¼ tbsp. Worcestershire sauce
- ½ tsp. olive oil
- ½ flake garlic crushed
- ¼ cup chopped onion
- ¼ tsp. mustard powder
- 1 tbsp. tomato ketchup
- ½ tbsp. sugar
- ¼ tbsp. red chili sauce
- ½ cup water.
- A pinch of salt and black pepper to taste

Directions:

1. Take the slices of bread and remove the edges. Now cut the slices horizontally. Cook the ingredients for the sauce and wait till it thickens. Now, add the oyster to the sauce and stir till it obtains the flavors.
2. Roast the capsicum and peel the skin off. Cut the capsicum into slices. Mix the ingredients together and apply it to the bread slices. Pre-heat the oven for 5 minutes at 300 Fahrenheit. Open the basket of the Fryer and place the prepared Classic Sandwiches in it such that no two Classic Sandwiches are touching each other. Now keep the fryer at 250 degrees for around 15 minutes.
3. Turn the Classic Sandwiches in between the cooking process to cook both slices. Serve the Classic Sandwiches with tomato ketchup or mint sauce.

223.Herbed Salmon With Asparagus

Servings: 2

Cooking Time: 12 Minutes

Ingredients:

- 2 teaspoons olive oil, plus additional for drizzling
- 2 (5-ounce / 142-g) salmon fillets, with skin

- Salt and freshly ground black pepper, to taste
- 1 bunch asparagus, trimmed
- 1 teaspoon dried tarragon
- 1 teaspoon dried chives
- Fresh lemon wedges, for serving

Directions:

1. Rub the olive oil all over the salmon fillets. Sprinkle with salt and pepper to taste.
2. Put the asparagus on the foil-lined baking pan and place the salmon fillets on top, skin-side down.
3. Slide the baking pan into Rack Position 1, select Convection Bake, set temperature to 350ºF (180ºC), and set time to 12 minutes.
4. When cooked, the fillets should register 145ºF (63ºC) on an instant-read thermometer. Remove from the oven and cut the salmon fillets in half crosswise, then use a metal spatula to lift flesh from skin and transfer to a serving plate. Discard the skin and drizzle the salmon fillets with additional olive oil. Scatter with the herbs.
5. Serve the salmon fillets with asparagus spears and lemon wedges on the side.

224.Baked Pesto Salmon

Servings: 4
Cooking Time: 15 Minutes
Ingredients:

- 4 salmon fillets
- 1/3 cup parmesan cheese, grated
- 1/3 cup breadcrumbs
- 6 tbsp pesto

Directions:

1. Fit the oven with the rack in position
2. Place fish fillets into the baking dish.
3. Pour pesto over fish fillets.
4. Mix together breadcrumbs and parmesan cheese and sprinkle over fish.
5. Set to bake at 325 F for 20 minutes. After 5 minutes place the baking dish in the preheated oven.
6. Serve and enjoy.

- **Nutrition Info:** Calories 396 Fat 22.8 g Carbohydrates 8.3 g Sugar 2.1 g Protein 40.4 g Cholesterol 89 mg

225.Lemon-garlic Butter Lobster

Servings: 2
Cooking Time: 15 Minutes
Ingredients:

- 4 oz lobster tails
- 1 tsp garlic, minced
- 1 tbsp butter
- Salt and black pepper to taste
- ½ tbsp lemon Juice

Directions:

1. Add all the ingredients to a food processor except for lobster and blend well. Wash lobster and halve using a meat knife; clean the skin of the lobster and cover with the marinade.
2. Preheat your to 380 F on Air Fry function. Place the lobster in the cooking basket and fit in the baking tray; cook for 10 minutes. Serve with fresh herbs.

226.Chili Tuna Casserole

Servings:4
Cooking Time: 16 Minutes
Ingredients:

- ½ tablespoon sesame oil
- 1/3 cup yellow onions, chopped
- ½ bell pepper, deveined and chopped
- 2 cups canned tuna, chopped
- Cooking spray
- 5 eggs, beaten
- ½ chili pepper, deveined and finely minced
- 1½ tablespoons sour cream
- 1/3 teaspoon dried basil
- 1/3 teaspoon dried oregano
- Fine sea salt and ground black pepper, to taste

Directions:

1. Heat the sesame oil in a nonstick skillet over medium heat until it shimmers.
2. Add the onions and bell pepper and sauté for 4 minutes, stirring occasionally, or until tender.
3. Add the canned tuna and keep stirring until the tuna is heated through.
4. Meanwhile, coat the baking pan lightly with cooking spray.

5. Transfer the tuna mixture to the baking pan, along with the beaten eggs, chili pepper, sour cream, basil, and oregano. Stir to combine well. Season with sea salt and black pepper.
6. Slide the baking pan into Rack Position 1, select Convection Bake, set temperature to 325ºF (160ºC), and set time to 12 minutes.
7. When cooking is complete, the eggs should be completely set and the top lightly browned. Remove from the oven and serve on a plate.

227.Lemon Pepper Tilapia Fillets

Servings:4
Cooking Time: 15 Minutes
Ingredients:

- 1 lb tilapia fillets
- 1 tbsp Italian seasoning
- 2 tbsp canola oil
- 2 tbsp lemon pepper
- Salt to taste
- 2-3 butter buds

Directions:

1. Preheat your oven to 400 F on Bake function. Drizzle tilapia fillets with canola oil. In a bowl, mix salt, lemon pepper, butter buds, and Italian seasoning; spread on the fish. Place the fillet on a baking tray and press Start. Cook for 10 minutes until tender and crispy. Serve warm.

228.Tender & Juicy Cajun Cod

Servings: 6
Cooking Time: 15 Minutes
Ingredients:

- 3 cod fillets, cut in half
- 1 tbsp Cajun seasoning
- 1 tbsp garlic, minced
- 1 tbsp olive oil
- 1/4 cup butter, melted
- Pepper
- Salt

Directions:

1. Fit the oven with the rack in position
2. Season fish fillets with pepper and salt and place in a 9*13-inch baking dish.
3. Mix together the remaining ingredients and pour over fish fillets.
4. Set to bake at 400 F for 20 minutes. After 5 minutes place the baking dish in the preheated oven.
5. Serve and enjoy.

- **Nutrition Info:** Calories 126 Fat 10.4 g Carbohydrates 0.5 g Sugar 0 g Protein 8.2 g Cholesterol 42 mg

229.Glazed Tuna And Fruit Kebabs

Servings:4
Cooking Time: 10 Minutes
Ingredients:

- Kebabs:
- 1 pound (454 g) tuna steaks, cut into 1-inch cubes
- ½ cup canned pineapple chunks, drained, juice reserved
- ½ cup large red grapes
- Marinade:
- 1 tablespoon honey
- 1 teaspoon olive oil
- 2 teaspoons grated fresh ginger
- Pinch cayenne pepper
- Special Equipment:
- 4 metal skewers

Directions:

1. Make the kebabs: Thread, alternating tuna cubes, pineapple chunks, and red grapes, onto the metal skewers.
2. Make the marinade: Whisk together the honey, olive oil, ginger, and cayenne pepper in a small bowl. Brush generously the marinade over the kebabs and allow to sit for 10 minutes.
3. When ready, transfer the kebabs to the air fryer basket.
4. Put the air fryer basket on the baking pan and slide into Rack Position 2, select Air Fry, set temperature to 370ºF (188ºC), and set time to 10 minutes.
5. After 5 minutes, remove from the oven and flip the kebabs and brush with the remaining marinade. Return the pan to the oven and continue cooking for an additional 5 minutes.

6. When cooking is complete, the kebabs should reach an internal temperature of 145ºF (63ºC) on a meat thermometer. Remove from the oven and discard any remaining marinade. Serve hot.

230.Easy Baked Fish Fillet

Servings: 4
Cooking Time: 15 Minutes
Ingredients:

- 1 lb white fish fillets
- 2 tbsp dried parsley
- 1/4 tsp red chili flakes
- 2 tbsp garlic, minced
- 2 tbsp olive oil
- Pepper
- Salt

Directions:

1. Fit the oven with the rack in position
2. Place fish fillets in a baking dish and drizzle with oil.
3. Sprinkle with chili flakes, parsley, and garlic. Season with pepper and salt.
4. Set to bake at 400 F for 20 minutes. After 5 minutes place the baking dish in the preheated oven.
5. Serve and enjoy.

- **Nutrition Info:** Calories 262 Fat 15.6 g Carbohydrates 1.5 g Sugar 0.1 g Protein 28.1 g Cholesterol 87 mg

231.Delicious Fried Seafood

Servings: 4
Cooking Time: 15 Minutes
Ingredients:

- 1 lb fresh scallops, mussels, fish fillets, prawns, shrimp
- 2 eggs, lightly beaten
- Salt and black pepper to taste
- 1 cup breadcrumbs mixed with zest of 1 lemon

Directions:

1. Dip each piece of the seafood into the eggs and season with salt and pepper. Coat in the crumbs and spray with oil. Arrange into the frying basket and fit in the baking tray; cook for 10 minutes at 400 F on Air Fry function, turning once halfway through. Serve.

232.Quick Tuna Patties

Servings: 10
Cooking Time: 10 Minutes
Ingredients:

- 15 oz can tuna, drained and flaked
- 3 tbsp parmesan cheese, grated
- 1/2 cup breadcrumbs
- 1 tbsp lemon juice
- 2 eggs, lightly beaten
- 1/2 tsp dried mixed herbs
- 1/2 tsp garlic powder
- 2 tbsp onion, minced
- 1 celery stalk, chopped
- Pepper
- Salt

Directions:

1. Fit the oven with the rack in position 2.
2. Add all ingredients into the mixing bowl and mix until well combined.
3. Make patties from mixture and place in the air fryer basket then place the air fryer basket in the baking pan.
4. Place a baking pan on the oven rack. Set to air fry at 360 F for 10 minutes.
5. Serve and enjoy.

- **Nutrition Info:** Calories 90 Fat 1.8 g Carbohydrates 4.4 g Sugar 0.6 g Protein 13.2 g Cholesterol 47 mg

233.Citrus Cilantro Catfish

Servings:2
Cooking Time: 20 Minutes
Ingredients:

- 2 catfish fillets
- 2 tsp blackening seasoning
- Juice of 1 lime
- 2 tbsp butter, melted
- 1 garlic clove, mashed
- 2 tbsp fresh cilantro, chopped

Directions:

1. In a bowl, blend garlic, lime juice, cilantro, and butter. Pour half of the mixture over the fillets and sprinkle with blackening seasoning. Place the fillets in the basket and press Start. Cook for 15 minutes at 360 F on AirFry function. Serve the fish topped with the remaining sauce.

234.Spicy Lemon Cod

Servings: 2

Cooking Time: 10 Minutes

Ingredients:

- 1 lb cod fillets
- 1/4 tsp chili powder
- 1 tbsp fresh parsley, chopped
- 1 1/2 tbsp olive oil
- 1 tbsp fresh lemon juice
- 1/8 tsp cayenne pepper
- 1/4 tsp salt

Directions:

1. Fit the oven with the rack in position
2. Arrange fish fillets in a baking dish. Drizzle with oil and lemon juice.
3. Sprinkle with chili powder, salt, and cayenne pepper.
4. Set to bake at 400 F for 15 minutes. After 5 minutes place the baking dish in the preheated oven.
5. Garnish with parsley and serve.

- **Nutrition Info:** Calories 276 Fat 12.7 g Carbohydrates 0.5 g Sugar 0.2 g Protein 40.7 g Cholesterol 111 mg

MEATLESS RECIPES

235.Banana Best Homemade Croquette

Servings:x

Cooking Time:x

Ingredients:

- 2 tsp. garam masala
- 4 tbsp. chopped coriander
- 3 tbsp. cream
- 3 tbsp. chopped capsicum
- 3 eggs
- 2 ½ tbsp. white sesame seeds
- 2 cups sliced banana
- 3 onions chopped
- 5 green chilies-roughly chopped
- 1 ½ tbsp. ginger paste
- 1 ½ tsp. garlic paste
- 1 ½ tsp. salt
- 3 tsp. lemon juice

Directions:

1. Grind the ingredients except for the egg and form a smooth paste. Coat the banana in the paste. Now, beat the eggs and add a little salt to it.
2. Dip the coated bananas in the egg mixture and then transfer to the sesame seeds and coat the vegetables well. Place the vegetables on a stick.
3. Pre heat the oven at 160 degrees Fahrenheit for around 5 minutes. Place the sticks in the basket and let them cook for another 25 minutes at the same temperature. Turn the sticks over in between the cooking process to get a uniform cook.

236.Asian Tofu "meatballs"

Servings: 4

Cooking Time: 10 Minutes

Ingredients:

- 3 dried shitake mushrooms
- Nonstick cooking spray
- 14 oz. firm tofu, drained & pressed
- ¼ cup carrots, cooked
- ¼ cup bamboo shoots, sliced thin
- ½ cup Panko bread crumbs
- 2 tbsp. corn starch
- 3 ½ tablespoon soy sauce, divided
- 1 tsp garlic powder
- ¼ tsp salt
- 1/8 tsp pepper
- 1 tbsp. olive oil
- 2 tbsp. garlic, diced fine
- 2 tbsp. ketchup
- 2 tsp sugar

Directions:

1. Place the shitake mushrooms in a bowl and add just enough water to cover. Let soak 20 minutes until soft. Drain well and chop.
2. Place the baking pan in position Lightly spray the fryer basket with cooking spray.
3. Place mushrooms, tofu, carrots, bamboo shoots, bread crumbs, corn starch, 1 ½ tablespoons soy sauce, and seasonings in a food processor. Pulse until thoroughly combined. Form mixture into 1-inch balls.
4. Place balls in fryer basket, these may need to be cooked in batches, and place in oven. Set to air fry on 380°F for 10 minutes. Turn the balls around halfway through cooking time.
5. Heat oil in a saucepan over medium heat. Add garlic and cook 1 minute.
6. Stir in remaining soy sauce, ketchup, and sugar. Bring to a simmer and cook until sauce thickens, 3-5 minutes.
7. When the meatballs are done, add them to sauce and stir to coat. Serve immediately.

- **Nutrition Info:** Calories 305, Total Fat 13g, Saturated Fat 2g, Total Carbs 28g, Net Carbs 24g, Protein 20g, Sugar 5g, Fiber 4g, Sodium 789mg, Potassium 470mg, Phosphorus 260mg

237.Cheese And Bean Enchiladas

Servings:x

Cooking Time:x

Ingredients:

- A pinch of salt or to taste
- A few red chili flakes to sprinkle
- 1 tsp. of oregano
- 2 tbsp. oil
- 2 tsp. chopped garlic

- 2 onions chopped finely
- 2 capsicums chopped finely
- 2 cups of readymade baked beans
- Flour tortillas (as many as required)
- 4 tbsp. of olive oil
- A pinch of salt
- 1 tsp. oregano
- ½ tsp. pepper
- 1 ½ tsp. red chili flakes or to taste
- 1 tbsp. of finely chopped jalapenos
- 1 cup grated pizza cheese (mix mozzarella and cheddar cheeses)
- 1 ½ tsp. of garlic that has been chopped
- 1 ½ cups of readymade tomato puree
- 3 medium tomatoes. Puree them in a mixer
- 1 tsp. of sugar
- A few drops of Tabasco sauce
- 1 cup crumbled or roughly mashed cottage cheese (cottage cheese)
- 1 cup grated cheddar cheese

Directions:

1. Prepare the flour tortillas. Now move on to making the red sauce. In a pan, pour around 2 tbsp. of oil and heat. Add some garlic. Add the rest of the ingredients mentioned under the heading "For the sauce".
2. Keep stirring. Cook until the sauce reduces and becomes thick. For the filling, heat one tbsp. of oil in another pan. Add onions and garlic and cook until the onions are caramelized or attain a golden-brown color. Add the rest of the ingredients required for the filling and cook for two to three minutes.
3. Take the pan off the flame and grate some cheese over the sauce. Mix it well and let it sit for a while. Let us start assembling the dish. Take a tortilla and spread some of the sauce on the surface. Now place the filling at the center in a line. Roll up the tortilla carefully. Do the same for all the tortillas. Now place all the tortillas in a tray and sprinkle them with grated cheese. Cover this with an aluminum foil. Pre heat the oven at 160° C for 4-5 minutes. Open the basket and place the tray inside.
4. Keep the fryer at the same temperature for another 15 minutes. Turn the tortillas over in between to get a uniform cook.

238.Radish Flat Cakes

Servings:x

Cooking Time:x

Ingredients:

- 1-2 tbsp. fresh coriander leaves
- 2 or 3 green chilies finely chopped
- 1 ½ tbsp. lemon juice
- Salt and pepper to taste
- 2 tbsp. garam masala
- 2 cups sliced radish
- 3 tsp. ginger finely chopped

Directions:

1. Mix the ingredients in a clean bowl and add water to it. Make sure that the paste is not too watery but is enough to apply on the radish.
2. Pre heat the oven at 160 degrees Fahrenheit for 5 minutes. Place the French Cuisine Galettes in the fry basket and let them cook for another 25 minutes at the same temperature. Keep rolling them over to get a uniform cook. Serve either with mint sauce or ketchup.

239.Cabbage Fritters(2)

Servings:x

Cooking Time:x

Ingredients:

- 1 ½ tsp. salt
- 3 tsp. lemon juice
- 2 tsp. garam masala
- 3 eggs
- 2 ½ tbsp. white sesame seeds
- 10 leaves cabbage
- 3 onions chopped
- 5 green chilies-roughly chopped
- 1 ½ tbsp. ginger paste
- 1 ½ tsp. garlic paste

Directions:

1. Grind the ingredients except for the egg and form a smooth paste. Coat the leaves in the paste. Now, beat the eggs and add a little salt to it.
2. Dip the coated leaves in the egg mixture and then transfer to the sesame seeds and coat the florets well. Place the vegetables on a stick.

3. Pre heat the oven at 160 degrees Fahrenheit for around 5 minutes. Place the sticks in the basket and let them cook for another 25 minutes at the same temperature. Turn the sticks over in between the cooking process to get a uniform cook.

240.Mexican Burritos

Servings:x

Cooking Time:x

Ingredients:

- 1 tbsp. Olive oil
- 1 medium onion finely sliced
- 3 flakes garlic crushed
- 1 tsp. freshly ground peppercorns
- ½ cup pickled jalapenos (Chop them up finely)
- 2 carrots (Cut in to long thin slices)
- 1-2 lettuce leaves shredded.
- 1 or 2 spring onions chopped finely. Also cut the greens.
- Take one tomato. Remove the seeds and chop it into small pieces.
- ½ cup French beans (Slice them lengthwise into thin and long slices)
- ½ cup mushrooms thinly sliced
- 1 cup cottage cheese cut in too long and slightly thick Oregano Fingers
- ½ cup shredded cabbage
- 1 tbsp. coriander, chopped
- 1 tbsp. vinegar
- 1 tsp. white wine
- ½ cup red kidney beans (soaked overnight)
- ½ small onion chopped
- 1 tbsp. olive oil
- 2 tbsp. tomato puree
- ¼ tsp. red chili powder
- 1 tsp. of salt to taste
- 4-5 flour tortillas
- A pinch of salt to taste
- ½ tsp. red chili flakes
- 1 green chili chopped.
- 1 cup of cheddar cheese grated.

Directions:

1. Cook the beans along with the onion and garlic and mash them finely. Now, make the sauce you will need for the burrito. Ensure that you create a slightly thick sauce.
2. For the filling, you will need to cook the ingredients well in a pan and ensure that the vegetables have browned on the outside.
3. To make the salad, toss the ingredients together.

241.Tofu & Pea Cauli Rice

Servings:4

Cooking Time: 30 Minutes

Ingredients:

- Tofu:
- ½ block tofu
- ½ cup onions, chopped
- 2 tbsp soy sauce
- 1 tsp turmeric
- 1 cup carrots, chopped
- Cauliflower:
- 3 cups cauliflower rice
- 2 tbsp soy sauce
- ½ cup broccoli, chopped
- 2 garlic cloves, minced
- 1 ½ tsp toasted sesame oil
- 1 tbsp fresh ginger, minced
- ½ cup frozen peas
- 1 tbsp rice vinegar

Directions:

1. Preheat on AirFry function to 370 F. Crumble the tofu and combine it with all tofu ingredients. Place in a baking dish and cook for 10 minutes.
2. Meanwhile, place all cauliflower ingredients in a large bowl; mix to combine. Add the cauliflower mixture to the tofu and stir to combine. Press Start and cook for 12 minutes. Serve.

242.Cottage Cheese Pops

Servings:x

Cooking Time:x

Ingredients:

- 1 tsp. dry basil
- ½ cup hung curd
- 1 tsp. lemon juice
- 1 cup cottage cheese cut into 2" cubes
- 1 ½ tsp. garlic paste
- Salt and pepper to taste

- 1 tsp. dry oregano
- 1 tsp. red chili flakes

Directions:

1. Cut the cottage cheese into thick and long rectangular pieces.
2. Add the rest of the ingredients into a separate bowl and mix them well to get a consistent mixture.
3. Dip the cottage cheese pieces in the above mixture and leave them aside for some time.
4. Pre heat the oven at 180° C for around 5 minutes. Place the coated cottage cheese pieces in the fry basket and close it properly. Let them cook at the same temperature for 20 more minutes. Keep turning them over in the basket so that they are cooked properly. Serve with tomato ketchup.

243.Crispy Eggplant Slices With Parsley

Servings:4

Cooking Time: 12 Minutes

Ingredients:

- 1 cup flour
- 4 eggs
- Salt, to taste
- 2 cups bread crumbs
- 1 teaspoon Italian seasoning
- 2 eggplants, sliced
- 2 garlic cloves, sliced
- 2 tablespoons chopped parsley
- Cooking spray

Directions:

1. Spritz the air fryer basket with cooking spray. Set aside.
2. On a plate, place the flour. In a shallow bowl, whisk the eggs with salt. In another shallow bowl, combine the bread crumbs and Italian seasoning.
3. Dredge the eggplant slices, one at a time, in the flour, then in the whisked eggs, finally in the bread crumb mixture to coat well.
4. Lay the coated eggplant slices in the basket.
5. Put the air fryer basket on the baking pan and slide into Rack Position 2, select Air Fry, set temperature to 390ºF (199ºC), and set time to 12 minutes.
6. Flip the eggplant slices halfway through the cooking time.
7. When cooking is complete, the eggplant slices should be golden brown and crispy. Transfer the eggplant slices to a plate and sprinkle the garlic and parsley on top before serving.

244.Veggie Delight

Servings:2

Cooking Time: 30 Minutes

Ingredients:

- 1 parsnip, sliced in a 2-inch thickness
- 1 cup chopped butternut squash
- 2 small red onions, cut in wedges
- 1 cup celery, chopped
- 1 tbsp fresh thyme, chopped
- Salt and black pepper to taste
- 2 tsp olive oil

Directions:

1. Preheat on AirFry function to 350 F. In a bowl, add turnip, squash, red onions, celery, thyme, pepper, salt, and olive oil and mix well. Add the veggies to the frying basket and press Start. Cook for 16 minutes, tossing once halfway through. Serve warm.

245.Classic Ratatouille

Servings: 2

Cooking Time: 30 Minutes

Ingredients:

- 1 tbsp olive oil
- 3 roma tomatoes, thinly sliced
- 2 garlic cloves, minced
- 1 zucchini, thinly sliced
- 2 yellow bell peppers, sliced
- 1 tbsp red wine vinegar
- 2 tbsp herbs de Provence
- Salt and black pepper to taste

Directions:

1. Preheat on Air Fry function to 390 F. In a bowl, mix together olive oil, garlic, vinegar, herbs, salt, and pepper. Add in tomatoes, zucchini, and bell peppers and toss to coat.
2. Arrange the vegetables in a baking dish and cook for 15 minutes, shaking occasionally. Let sit for 5 more minutes after the timer goes off. Serve.

246.Winter Vegetarian Frittata

Servings: 4
Cooking Time: 30 Minutes
Ingredients:

- 1 leek, peeled and thinly sliced into rings
- 2 cloves garlic, finely minced
- 3 medium-sized carrots, finely chopped
- 2 tablespoons olive oil
- 6 large-sized eggs
- Sea salt and ground black pepper, to taste
- 1/2 teaspoon dried marjoram, finely minced
- 1/2 cup yellow cheese of choice

Directions:

1. Preparing the Ingredients. Sauté the leek, garlic, and carrot in hot olive oil until they are tender and fragrant; reserve.
2. In the meantime, preheat your air fryer oven to 330 degrees F.
3. In a bowl, whisk the eggs along with the salt, ground black pepper, and marjoram.
4. Then, grease the inside of your baking dish with a nonstick cooking spray. Pour the whisked eggs into the baking dish. Stir in the sautéed carrot mixture. Top with the cheese shreds.
5. Air Frying. Place the baking dish in the air fryer oven cooking basket. Cook about 30 minutes and serve warm

247.Mushroom Wonton

Servings:x
Cooking Time:x
Ingredients:

- 2 cups cubed mushroom
- 2 tbsp. oil
- 2 tsp. ginger-garlic paste
- 2 tsp. soya sauce
- 2 tsp. vinegar
- 1 ½ cup all-purpose flour
- ½ tsp. salt or to taste
- 5 tbsp. water

Directions:

1. Squeeze the dough and cover it with plastic wrap and set aside. Next, cook the ingredients for the filling and try to ensure that the mushroom is covered well with the sauce.
2. Roll the dough and place the filling in the center. Now, wrap the dough to cover the filling and pinch the edges together.
3. Pre heat the oven at 200° F for 5 minutes. Place the dumplings in the fry basket and close it. Let them cook at the same temperature for another 20 minutes. Recommended sides are chili sauce or ketchup.

248.Chinese Spring Rolls

Servings:4
Cooking Time: 15 Minutes
Ingredients:

- ½ head cabbage, grated
- 2 carrots, grated
- 1 tsp fresh ginger, minced
- 1 garlic clove, minced
- 1 tsp sesame oil
- 1 tsp soy sauce
- 1 tsp sesame seeds
- ½ tsp salt
- 1 tsp olive oil
- 1 package spring roll wrappers

Directions:

1. Combine all ingredients in a bowl. Divide the mixture between the roll sheets and roll them up; arrange on a baking tray. Press Start and cook in the for 5 minutes on Bake function at 370 F.

249.Cauliflower French Cuisine Galette

Servings:x
Cooking Time:x
Ingredients:

- 3 tsp. ginger finely chopped
- 1-2 tbsp. fresh coriander leaves
- 2 or 3 green chilies finely chopped
- 1 ½ tbsp. lemon juice
- Salt and pepper to taste
- 2 tbsp. garam masala
- 2 cups cauliflower
- 1 ½ cup coarsely crushed peanuts

Directions:

1. Mix the ingredients in a clean bowl.

2. Mold this mixture into round and flat French Cuisine Galettes.
3. Wet the French Cuisine Galettes slightly with water. Coat each French Cuisine Galette with the crushed peanuts.
4. Pre heat the oven at 160 degrees Fahrenheit for 5 minutes. Place the French Cuisine Galettes in the fry basket and let them cook for another 25 minutes at the same temperature. Keep rolling them over to get a uniform cook. Serve either with mint sauce or ketchup.

250.Garlic Toast With Cheese

Servings:x
Cooking Time:x
Ingredients:

- ¾ cup grated cheese
- 2 tsp. of oregano seasoning
- Some red chili flakes to sprinkle on top
- Take some French bread and cut it into slices
- 1 tbsp. olive oil (Optional)
- 2 tbsp. softened butter
- 4-5 flakes crushed garlic
- A pinch of salt to taste
- ½ tsp. black pepper powder

Directions:

1. Take a clean and dry container. Place all the ingredients mentioned under the heading "Garlic Butter" into it and mix properly to obtain garlic butter. On each slice of the French bread, spread some of this garlic butter. Sprinkle some cheese on top of the layer of butter. Pour some oil if wanted.
2. Sprinkle some chili flakes and some oregano.
3. Pre heat the oven at 240 Fahrenheit for around 5 minutes. Open the fry basket and place the bread in it making sure that no two slices touch each other. Close the basket and continue to cook the bread at 160 degrees for another 10 minutes to toast the bread well.

251.Herby Tofu

Servings: 2
Cooking Time: 30 Minutes
Ingredients:

- 6 oz extra firm tofu
- Black pepper to taste
- 1 tbsp vegetable broth
- 1 tbsp soy sauce
- ⅓ tsp dried oregano
- ⅓ tsp garlic powder
- ⅓ tsp dried basil
- ⅓ tsp onion powder

Directions:

1. Place the tofu on a cutting board and cut it into 3 lengthwise slices with a knife. Line a side of the cutting board with paper towels, place the tofu on it, and cover with a paper towel. Use your hands to press the tofu gently until as much liquid has been extracted from it. Chop the tofu into 8 cubes; set aside.
2. In another bowl, add the soy sauce, vegetable broth, oregano, basil, garlic powder, onion powder, and black pepper and mix well with a spoon. Rub the spice mixture on the tofu. Let it marinate for 10 minutes.
3. Preheat on Air Fry function to 390 F. Place the tofu in the fryer's basket in a single layer and fit in the baking tray. Cook for 10 minutes, flipping it at the 6-minute mark. Remove to a plate and serve with green salad.

252.Herbed Broccoli With Cheese

Servings:4
Cooking Time: 18 Minutes
Ingredients:

- 1 large-sized head broccoli, stemmed and cut into small florets
- 2½ tablespoons canola oil
- 2 teaspoons dried basil
- 2 teaspoons dried rosemary
- Salt and ground black pepper, to taste
- $^{1}/_{3}$ cup grated yellow cheese

Directions:

1. Bring a pot of lightly salted water to a boil. Add the broccoli florets to the boiling water and let boil for about 3 minutes.
2. Drain the broccoli florets well and transfer to a large bowl. Add the canola oil, basil,

rosemary, salt, and black pepper to the bowl and toss until the broccoli is fully coated. Place the broccoli in the air fryer basket.

3. Put the air fryer basket on the baking pan and slide into Rack Position 2, select Air Fry, set temperature to 390ºF (199ºC), and set time to 15 minutes.
4. Stir the broccoli halfway through the cooking time.
5. When cooking is complete, the broccoli should be crisp. Serve the broccoli warm with grated cheese sprinkled on top.

253.Roasted Vegetable Mélange With Herbs

Servings:4

Cooking Time: 16 Minutes

Ingredients:

- 1 (8-ounce / 227-g) package sliced mushrooms
- 1 yellow summer squash, sliced
- 1 red bell pepper, sliced
- 3 cloves garlic, sliced
- 1 tablespoon olive oil
- ½ teaspoon dried basil
- ½ teaspoon dried thyme
- ½ teaspoon dried tarragon

Directions:

1. Toss the mushrooms, squash, and bell pepper with the garlic and olive oil in a large bowl until well coated. Mix in the basil, thyme, and tarragon and toss again.
2. Spread the vegetables evenly in the air fryer basket.
3. Put the air fryer basket on the baking pan and slide into Rack Position 2, select Roast, set temperature to 350ºF (180ºC), and set time to 16 minutes.
4. When cooking is complete, the vegetables should be fork-tender. Remove from the oven and cool for 5 minutes before serving.

254.Simple Polenta Crisps

Servings:4

Cooking Time: 25 Minutes + Chilling Time

Ingredients:

- 2 cups milk
- 1 cup instant polenta
- Salt and black pepper
- Fresh thyme, chopped

Directions:

1. Line a tray with parchment paper. Pour milk and 2 cups of water into a saucepan and simmer. Keep whisking as you pour in the polenta. Continue to whisk until polenta thickens and bubbles; season to taste. Add polenta to the lined tray and spread out. Refrigerate for 45 minutes.
2. Slice the polenta into batons and spray with oil. Arrange the polenta chips on the basket and press Start. Cook for 16 minutes at 380 F on AirFry function until golden and crispy.

255.Rosemary Roasted Squash With Cheese

Servings:2

Cooking Time: 20 Minutes

Ingredients:

- 1 pound (454 g) butternut squash, cut into wedges
- 2 tablespoons olive oil
- 1 tablespoon dried rosemary
- Salt, to salt
- 1 cup crumbled goat cheese
- 1 tablespoon maple syrup

Directions:

1. Toss the squash wedges with the olive oil, rosemary, and salt in a large bowl until well coated.
2. Transfer the squash wedges to the air fryer basket, spreading them out in as even a layer as possible.
3. Put the air fryer basket on the baking pan and slide into Rack Position 2, select Air Fry, set temperature to 350ºF (180ºC), and set time to 20 minutes.
4. After 10 minutes, remove from the oven and flip the squash. Return the pan to the oven and continue cooking for 10 minutes.
5. When cooking is complete, the squash should be golden brown. Remove from the oven. Sprinkle the goat cheese on top and serve drizzled with the maple syrup.

256.Honey Chili Potatoes

Servings:x
Cooking Time:x
Ingredients:

- 1 capsicum, cut into thin and long pieces (lengthwise).
- 2 tbsp. olive oil
- 2 onions. Cut them into halves.
- 1 ½ tbsp. sweet chili sauce
- 1 ½ tsp. ginger garlic paste
- ½ tbsp. red chili sauce.
- 2 tbsp. tomato ketchup
- 3 big potatoes (Cut into strips or cubes)
- 2 ½ tsp. ginger-garlic paste
- ¼ tsp. salt
- 1 tsp. red chili sauce
- ¼ tsp. red chili powder/black pepper
- A few drops of edible orange food coloring
- 2 tsp. soya sauce
- 2 tsp. vinegar
- A pinch of black pepper powder
- 1-2 tsp. red chili flakes

Directions:

1. Create the mix for the potato Oregano Fingers and coat the chicken well with it.
2. Pre heat the oven at 250 Fahrenheit for 5 minutes or so. Open the basket of the Fryer. Place the Oregano Fingers inside the basket. Now let the fryer stay at 290 Fahrenheit for another 20 minutes. Keep tossing the Oregano Fingers periodically through the cook to get a uniform cook.
3. Add the ingredients to the sauce and cook it with the vegetables till it thickens. Add the Oregano Fingers to the sauce and cook till the flavors have blended.

257.Nutmeg Broccoli With Eggs & Cheddar Cheese

Servings:4
Cooking Time: 15 Minutes
Ingredients:

- 1 lb broccoli, cut into florets
- 4 eggs
- 1 cup cheddar cheese, shredded
- 1 cup heavy cream
- 1 pinch of nutmeg
- 1 tsp ginger powder

Directions:

1. In boiling water, steam the broccoli for 5 minutes. Drain and place in a bowl. Add in 1 egg, heavy cream, nutmeg, and ginger. Divide the mixture between greased ramekins and sprinkle the cheddar cheese on top. Cook for 10 minutes at 280 F on AirFry function.

258.Feta & Scallion Triangles

Servings:4
Cooking Time: 20 Minutes
Ingredients:

- 4 oz feta cheese, crumbled
- 2 sheets filo pastry
- 1 egg yolk, beaten
- 2 tbsp fresh parsley, finely chopped
- 1 scallion, finely chopped
- 2 tbsp olive oil
- Salt and black pepper to taste

Directions:

1. In a bowl, mix the yolk with the cheese, parsley, and scallion. Season with salt and black pepper. Cut each filo sheet in 3 strips. Put a teaspoon of the feta mixture on the bottom. Roll the strip in a spinning spiral way until the filling of the inside mixture is completely wrapped in a triangle.
2. Preheat on Bake function to 360 F. Brush the surface of filo with olive oil. Place up to 5 triangles in the oven and press Start. Cook for 5 minutes. Lower the temperature to 330 F, cook for 3 more minutes or until golden brown.

259.Tofu, Carrot And Cauliflower Rice

Servings:4
Cooking Time: 22 Minutes
Ingredients:

- ½ block tofu, crumbled
- 1 cup diced carrot
- ½ cup diced onions
- 2 tablespoons soy sauce
- 1 teaspoon turmeric
- Cauliflower:
- 3 cups cauliflower rice
- ½ cup chopped broccoli

- ½ cup frozen peas
- 2 tablespoons soy sauce
- 1 tablespoon minced ginger
- 2 garlic cloves, minced
- 1 tablespoon rice vinegar
- 1½ teaspoons toasted sesame oil

Directions:

1. Mix the tofu, carrot, onions, soy sauce, and turmeric in a baking pan and stir until well incorporated.
2. Slide the baking pan into Rack Position 2, select Roast, set temperature to 370ºF (188ºC) and set time to 10 minutes.
3. Flip the tofu and carrot halfway through the cooking time.
4. When cooking is complete, the tofu should be crisp.
5. Meanwhile, in a large bowl, combine all the ingredients for the cauliflower and toss well.
6. Remove the pan from the oven and add the cauliflower mixture to the tofu and stir to combine.
7. Return to the oven and set time to 12 minutes on Roast.
8. When cooking is complete, the vegetables should be tender.
9. Cool for 5 minutes before serving.

260.Spicy Sweet Potato Friespotato Fries

Servings: 4
Cooking Time: 37 Minutes
Ingredients:

- 2 tbsp. sweet potato fry seasoning mix
- 2 tbsp. olive oil
- 2 sweet potatoes
- Seasoning Mix:
- 2 tbsp. salt
- 1 tbsp. cayenne pepper
- 1 tbsp. dried oregano
- 1 tbsp. fennel
- 2 tbsp. coriander

Directions:

1. Preparing the Ingredients. Slice both ends off sweet potatoes and peel. Slice lengthwise in half and again crosswise to make four pieces from each potato.
2. Slice each potato piece into 2-3 slices, then slice into fries.
3. Grind together all of seasoning mix ingredients and mix in the salt.
4. Ensure the air fryer oven is preheated to 350 degrees.
5. Toss potato pieces in olive oil, sprinkling with seasoning mix and tossing well to coat thoroughly.
6. Air Frying. Add fries to air fryer rack/basket. Set temperature to 350°F, and set time to 27 minutes. Select START/STOP to begin.
7. Take out the basket and turn fries. Turn off air fryer oven and let cook 10-12 minutes till fries are golden.

- **Nutrition Info:** CALORIES: 89; FAT: 14G; PROTEIN: 8Gs; SUGAR:3

261.Bottle Gourd Flat Cakes

Servings:x
Cooking Time:x
Ingredients:

- 2 or 3 green chilies finely chopped
- 1 ½ tbsp. lemon juice
- Salt and pepper to taste
- 2 tbsp. garam masala
- 2 cups sliced bottle gourd
- 3 tsp. ginger finely chopped
- 1-2 tbsp. fresh coriander leaves

Directions:

1. Mix the ingredients in a clean bowl and add water to it. Make sure that the paste is not too watery but is enough to apply on the bottle gourd slices. Pre heat the oven at 160 degrees Fahrenheit for 5 minutes.
2. Place the French Cuisine Galettes in the fry basket and let them cook for another 25 minutes at the same temperature. Keep rolling them over to get a uniform cook. Serve either with mint sauce or ketchup.

262.Garlicky Fennel Cabbage Steaks

Servings: 3
Cooking Time: 25 Minutes
Ingredients:

- 1 cabbage head
- 1 tbsp garlic paste
- 1 tsp salt
- 2 tbsp olive oil
- ½ tsp black pepper

- 2 tsp fennel seeds

Directions:

1. Preheat on Air Fry function to 350 F. Slice the cabbage into 1 ½-inch slices. In a small bowl, combine all the other ingredients; brush cabbage with the mixture. Arrange the steaks on a greased baking dish and cook for 15 minutes, flipping once. Serve.

263.Carrot & Chickpea Oat Balls With Cashews

Servings:4

Cooking Time: 30 Minutes

Ingredients:

- 2 tbsp olive oil
- 2 tbsp soy sauce
- 1 tbsp flax meal
- 2 cups canned chickpeas, drained
- ½ cup sweet onions, diced
- ½ cup carrots, grated
- ½ cup cashews, toasted
- Juice of 1 lemon
- ½ tsp turmeric
- 1 tsp cumin
- 1 tsp garlic powder
- 1 cup rolled oats

Directions:

1. Preheat on AirFry function to 380 F. Heat olive oil in a skillet and sauté onions and carrots for 5 minutes. Ground the oats and cashews in a food processor. Transfer to a bowl.
2. Place the chickpeas, lemon juice, and soy sauce in the food processor and process until smooth. Add them to the bowl as well. Mix in the onions and carrots.
3. Stir in the remaining ingredients until fully incorporated. Make balls out of the mixture. Place them in the frying basket and press Start. Cook for 12 minutes. Serve warm.

264.Broccoli & Cheese Egg Ramekins

Servings: 4

Cooking Time: 25 Minutes

Ingredients:

- 1 lb broccoli
- 4 eggs, beaten
- 1 cup cheddar cheese, shredded
- 1 cup heavy cream
- ½ tsp ground nutmeg
- 1 tsp ginger powder
- Salt and black pepper to taste

Directions:

1. In boiling water, steam the broccoli for 5 minutes. Drain and place in a bowl to cool. Mix in the eggs, heavy cream, nutmeg, ginger, salt, and pepper. Divide the mixture between greased ramekins and sprinkle the cheddar cheese on top. Place in a baking tray and cook in your for 10 minutes at 360 F on Bake function. Serve.

265.Mushroom Club Sandwich

Servings:x

Cooking Time:x

Ingredients:

- ¼ tbsp. Worcestershire sauce
- ½ tsp. olive oil
- ½ flake garlic crushed
- ¼ cup chopped onion
- ¼ tbsp. red chili sauce
- ½ cup water
- 2 slices of white bread
- 1 tbsp. softened butter
- 1 cup minced mushroom
- 1 small capsicum

Directions:

1. Take the slices of bread and remove the edges. Now cut the slices horizontally.
2. Cook the ingredients for the sauce and wait till it thickens. Now, add the mushroom to the sauce and stir till it obtains the flavors. Roast the capsicum and peel the skin off. Cut the capsicum into slices. Apply the sauce on the slices.
3. Pre-heat the oven for 5 minutes at 300 Fahrenheit. Open the basket of the Fryer and place the prepared Classic Sandwiches in it such that no two Classic Sandwiches are touching each other. Now keep the fryer at 250 degrees for around 15 minutes. Turn the Classic Sandwiches in between the cooking process to cook both slices. Serve the Classic Sandwiches with tomato ketchup or mint sauce.

266.Green Chili Taquitos

Servings: 3
Cooking Time: 10 Minutes
Ingredients:

- Nonstick cooking spray
- 6 corn tortillas
- ¾ cup vegan cream cheese
- 1 cup vegan cheddar cheese, grated
- 4 oz. green chilies, diced & drained

Directions:

1. Place baking pan in position 2. Lightly spray fryer basket with cooking spray.
2. Wrap tortillas in paper towels and microwave 1 minute.
3. Spread the cream cheese over tortillas. Top with cheddar cheese and chilies. Roll up tightly. Place, seam side down, in fryer basket.
4. Place the basket on the baking pan and set oven to air fry on 350°F for 10 minutes or until tortillas are browned and crispy. Turn taquitos over halfway through cooking time. Serve immediately.

- **Nutrition Info:** Calories 706, Total Fat 34g, Saturated Fat 18g, Total Carbs 51g, Net Carbs 35g, Protein 24g, Sugar 11g, Fiber 16g, Sodium 2371mg, Potassium 1074mg, Phosphorus 850mg

267.Cheesy Potato Wedges

Servings:x
Cooking Time:x
Ingredients:

- A pinch of salt to taste
- 1 tbsp. lemon juice
- 1 cup molten cheese
- 2 medium sized potatoes (Cut into wedges)
- ingredients for the marinade:
- 1 tbsp. olive oil
- 1 tsp. mixed herbs
- ½ tsp. red chili flakes

Directions:

1. Boil the potatoes and blanch them. Mix the ingredients for the marinade and add the potato Oregano Fingers to it making sure that they are coated well.
2. Pre heat the oven for around 5 minutes at 300 Fahrenheit. Take out the basket of the fryer and place the potato Oregano Fingers in them. Close the basket.
3. Now keep the fryer at 200 Fahrenheit for 20 or 25 minutes. In between the process, toss the fries twice or thrice so that they get cooked properly. Garnish with cheese and serve.

268.Masala French Cuisine Galette

Servings:x
Cooking Time:x
Ingredients:

- 1 ½ tbsp. lemon juice
- Salt and pepper to taste
- 1-2 tbsp. fresh coriander leaves
- 2 or 3 green chilies finely chopped
- 2 tbsp. garam masala
- 2 medium potatoes boiled and mashed
- 1 ½ cup coarsely crushed peanuts
- 3 tsp. ginger finely chopped

Directions:

1. Mix the ingredients in a clean bowl.
2. Mold this mixture into round and flat French Cuisine Galettes.
3. Wet the French Cuisine Galettes slightly with water. Coat each French Cuisine Galette with the crushed peanuts.
4. Pre heat the oven at 160 degrees Fahrenheit for 5 minutes. Place the French Cuisine Galettes in the fry basket and let them cook for another 25 minutes at the same temperature. Keep rolling them over to get a uniform cook. Serve either with mint sauce or ketchup.

269.Italian Baked Tofu

Servings:2
Cooking Time: 10 Minutes
Ingredients:

- 1 tablespoon soy sauce
- 1 tablespoon water
- $^{1}/_{3}$ teaspoon garlic powder
- $^{1}/_{3}$ teaspoon onion powder
- $^{1}/_{3}$ teaspoon dried oregano
- $^{1}/_{3}$ teaspoon dried basil
- Black pepper, to taste

- 6 ounces (170 g) extra firm tofu, pressed and cubed

Directions:

1. In a large mixing bowl, whisk together the soy sauce, water, garlic powder, onion powder, oregano, basil, and black pepper. Add the tofu cubes, stirring to coat, and let them marinate for 10 minutes.
2. Arrange the tofu in the baking pan.
3. Slide the baking pan into Rack Position 1, select Convection Bake, set temperature to 390ºF (199ºC) and set time to 10 minutes.
4. Flip the tofu halfway through the cooking time.
5. When cooking is complete, the tofu should be crisp.
6. Remove from the oven to a plate and serve.

270.Butter Burgers

Servings: 4

Cooking Time: 30 Minutes

Ingredients:

- Nonstick cooking spray
- ½ cup black beans, rinsed & drained
- 12 oz. mushrooms, sliced
- 1 ½ cup brown rice, cooked
- ½ cup oats
- 1 tsp salt
- ½ tsp pepper
- 1 tsp garlic powder
- 1 tsp onion powder
- ¼ tsp red pepper flakes
- ¼ cup Vegan butter
- 2 cups onions, sliced

Directions:

1. Place baking pan in position 2 in the oven. Lightly spray fryer basket with cooking spray.
2. Pat the beans with paper towel to get them as dry as possible.
3. Heat a medium skillet over med-high heat. Add mushrooms and cook, stirring frequently, until almost no moisture remains.
4. Add mushrooms, beans, rice, oats, and seasonings to a food processor. Pulse to chop and combine ingredients. Do not over blend. Let mixture rest 20 minutes.
5. Melt butter in a large skillet over medium heat. Add onions and cook until browned and tender.
6. Form mushroom mixture into 4 patties and place in the fryer basket. Place in oven and set to air fry on 350°F for 10 minutes. Cook burgers 8-10 minutes, until nicely browned, turning over halfway through cooking time.
7. Serve on toasted buns topped with cooked onions.

- **Nutrition Info:** Calories 351, Total Fat 15g, Saturated Fat 8g, Total Carbs 44g, Net Carbs 37g, Protein 10g, Sugar 4g, Fiber 7g, Sodium 704mg, Potassium 604mg, Phosphorus 286mg

271.Cheesy Cauliflower Fritters

Servings: 8

Cooking Time: 7 Minutes

Ingredients:

- ½ C. chopped parsley
- 1 C. Italian breadcrumbs
- 1/3 C. shredded mozzarella cheese
- 1/3 C. shredded sharp cheddar cheese
- 1 egg
- 2 minced garlic cloves
- 3 chopped scallions
- 1 head of cauliflower

Directions:

1. Preparing the Ingredients. Cut the cauliflower up into florets. Wash well and pat dry. Place into a food processor and pulse 20-30 seconds till it looks like rice.
2. Place cauliflower rice in a bowl and mix with pepper, salt, egg, cheeses, breadcrumbs, garlic, and scallions.
3. With hands, form 15 patties of the mixture. Add more breadcrumbs if needed.
4. Air Frying. With olive oil, spritz patties, and place into your air fryer oven in a single layer. Set temperature to 390°F, and set time to 7 minutes, flipping after 7 minutes.

- **Nutrition Info:** CALORIES: 209; FAT: 17G; PROTEIN: 6G; SUGAR:0.5

272.Amazing Macadamia Delight

Servings:6

Cooking Time: 20 Minutes

Ingredients:

- 3 cups macadamia nuts
- 3 tbsp liquid smoke
- Salt to taste
- 2 tbsp molasses

Directions:

1. Preheat on Bake function to 360 F. In a bowl, add salt, liquid, molasses, and cashews and toss to coat. Place the cashews ina baking tray and press Start. Cook for 10 minutes, shaking the basket every 5 minutes. Serve.

273.Caucasia Gnocchi's

Servings:x

Cooking Time:x

Ingredients:

- 2 cups minced colas Asia
- 2 tbsp. oil
- 2 tsp. ginger-garlic paste
- 2 tsp. soya sauce
- 2 tsp. vinegar
- 1 ½ cup all-purpose flour
- ½ tsp. salt
- 5 tbsp. water

Directions:

1. Squeeze the dough and cover it with plastic wrap and set aside. Next, cook the ingredients for the filling and try to ensure that the colas Asia is covered well with the sauce.
2. Roll the dough and place the filling in the center. Now, wrap the dough to cover the filling and pinch the edges together.
3. Pre heat the oven at 200° F for 5 minutes. Place the gnocchi's in the fry basket and close it. Let them cook at the same temperature for another 20 minutes. Recommended sides are chili sauce or ketchup.

274.Almond Cherry Bars

Servings: 12
Cooking Time: 35 Minutes
Ingredients:

- Xanthan gum, 1 tbsp.
- Almond flour, 1 ½ cup
- Salt, ½ tsp.
- Pitted fresh cherries, 1 cup
- Softened butter, ½ cup
- Eggs, 2.
- Water, ¼ cup
- Vanilla, ½ tsp.
- Erythritol, 1 cup

Directions:

1. Combine almond flour, softened butter, salt, vanilla, eggs, and erythritol in a large bowl until you form a dough.
2. Press the dough in a baking dish that will fit in the air fryer.
3. Set in the air fryer and bake for 10 minutes at 375 ºF
4. Meanwhile, mix the cherries, water, and xanthan gum in a bowl.
5. Take the dough out and pour over the cherry mixture.
6. Cook again for 25 minutes at 375 ºF in the air fryer.

- **Nutrition Info:** Calories: 99 Carbs: 2.1g Fat: 9.3g Protein: 1.8g

275.Quick Coffee Cake

Servings: 2
Cooking Time: 30 Minutes
Ingredients:

- ¼ cup butter
- ½ tsp instant coffee
- 1 tbsp black coffee, brewed
- 1 egg
- ¼ cup sugar
- ¼ cup flour
- 1 tsp cocoa powder
- Powdered sugar, for icing

Directions:

1. Preheat on Bake function to 330 F. Beat the sugar and egg together in a bowl. Beat in cocoa, instant and black coffees; stir in flour. Transfer the batter to a greased cake pan. Cook for 15 minutes. Dust with powdered sugar and serve.

276.Kale Chips With Sesame

Servings:5
Cooking Time: 8 Minutes
Ingredients:

- 8 cups deribbed kale leaves, torn into 2-inch pieces
- 1½ tablespoons olive oil
- ¾ teaspoon chili powder
- ¼ teaspoon garlic powder
- ½ teaspoon paprika
- 2 teaspoons sesame seeds

Directions:

1. In a large bowl, toss the kale with the olive oil, chili powder, garlic powder, paprika, and sesame seeds until well coated.
2. Transfer the kale to the air fryer basket.
3. Put the air fryer basket on the baking pan and slide into Rack Position 2, select Air Fry, set temperature to 350ºF (180ºC), and set time to 8 minutes.
4. Flip the kale twice during cooking.
5. When cooking is complete, the kale should be crispy. Remove from the oven and serve warm.

277.Simple Cinnamon Rolls

Servings: 8
Cooking Time: 10 Minutes
Ingredients:

- Nonstick cooking spray
- 1 tbsp. cinnamon
- ¾ stick butter, soft
- 6 tbsp. brown sugar
- 1 sheet puff pastry, thawed
- ½ cup powdered sugar
- 1 tbsp. milk
- 2 tsp fresh lemon juice

Directions:

1. Place baking pan in position 2. Lightly spray fryer basket with cooking spray.
2. In a small bowl, stir together cinnamon, butter, and sugar.

3. Gently roll out pastry and spread with cinnamon mixture covering it completely.
4. Carefully roll up the pastry, starting at the short end. Use a serrated knife to cut the pastry in 1-inch pieces.
5. Place them in the fryer basket, these will need to be cooked in 2 batches. Place the basket on the baking pan and set oven to air fry on 400°F for 8 minutes. Cook cinnamon rolls until puffed and golden brown. Repeat with remaining rolls.
6. Let cool slightly. In a small bowl, whisk together powdered sugar, milk, and lemon juice, drizzle over cinnamon rolls and serve.

- **Nutrition Info:** Calories 155, Total Fat 11g, Saturated Fat 6g, Total Carbs 13g, Net Carbs 12g, Protein 1g, Sugar 10g, Fiber 1g, Sodium 85mg, Potassium 19mg, Phosphorus 9mg

278.Chocolate Sponge Cake

Servings:x
Cooking Time:x
Ingredients:

- 3 tbsp. powdered sugar
- ½ cup soda
- 1 tsp. vanilla essence
- Parchment or butter paper to line the tin
- ½ cup condensed milk
- 1 cup all-purpose flour
- ½ cup cocoa powder
- ½ tsp. baking soda
- ½ tsp. baking powder
- ½ cup oil

Directions:

1. Mix the ingredients together to create a batter that is smooth and thick.
2. Grease a cake tin with butter and line it with the parchment or butter paper.
3. Transfer the batter into the tin.
4. Preheat the fryer to 300 Fahrenheit for five minutes. You will need to place the tin in the basket and cover it. Cook the cake for fifteen minutes and check whether or not the cake is cooked using a toothpick. Remove the tin and cut the cake into slices and serve.

279.Egg Rolls

Servings:x
Cooking Time:x
Ingredients:

- 1 cup shredded Napa cabbage
- 2 tablespoons soy sauce
- 1 tablespoon oyster sauce
- 2 tablespoons cornstarch 1 tablespoon water
- 1 package egg roll wrappers
- 3 cups peanut oil
- ½ pound ground pork
- ½ pound ground shrimp
- 1 carrot, shredded
- 2 cloves garlic, minced
- 1 bunch green onions, finely chopped

Directions:

1. In a large skillet, brown ground pork until almost done. Add ground shrimp, carrot, and garlic; cook and stir for 4 to 6 minutes or until pork is cooked. Remove from heat, drain well, and add green onions, cabbage, soy sauce, and oyster sauce.
2. Combine cornstarch and water in a small bowl and blend well.
3. To form egg rolls, place one wrapper, point-side down, on work surface. Place 1 tablespoon filling 1 inch from corner. Brush all edges of the egg roll wrapper with cornstarch mixture. Fold point over filling, then fold in sides and roll up egg roll, using cornstarch mixture to seal as necessary.
4. At this point, egg rolls may be flash frozen, or you can flash freeze them after frying. Once frozen, pack, label, and freeze in rigid containers.
5. To reheat untried egg rolls: Fry the frozen rolls in peanut oil heated to 375ºF for 2 to 3 minutes, turning once, or until deep golden brown. To reheat fried egg rolls: Place frozen egg rolls on baking sheet. Bake at 375ºF for 8 to 10 minutes or until crisp and hot.

280.Blackberry Crisp

Servings: 4
Cooking Time: 30 Minutes
Ingredients:

- 1 cup Crunchy Granola
- 2 cups blackberries
- ⅓ cup powdered erythritol
- 2 tbsp. lemon juice
- ¼ tsp. xanthan gum

Directions:

1. Take a large bowl, toss blackberries, erythritol, lemon juice and xanthan gum.
2. Pour into 6-inch round baking dish and cover with foil. Place into the air fryer basket.
3. Adjust the temperature to 350 Degrees F and set the timer for 12 minutes.
4. When the timer beeps, remove the foil and stir.
5. Sprinkle granola over mixture and return to the air fryer basket. Adjust the temperature to 320 Degrees F and set the timer for 3 minutes or until top is golden. Serve warm.

- **Nutrition Info:** Calories: 496; Protein: 9.2g; Fiber: 12.5g; Fat: 42.1g; Carbs: 44.0g

281.Delicious Jalapeno Poppers

Servings: 10
Cooking Time: 7 Minutes
Ingredients:

- 10 jalapeno peppers, cut in half, remove seeds & membranes
- 1/2 cup cheddar cheese, shredded
- 4 oz cream cheese
- 1/4 tsp paprika
- 1 tsp ground cumin
- 1 tsp salt

Directions:

1. Fit the oven with the rack in position 2.
2. In a small bowl, mix together cream cheese, cheddar cheese, cumin, paprika, and salt.
3. Stuff cream cheese mixture into each jalapeno half.
4. Place stuffed jalapeno peppers in air fryer basket then place air fryer basket in baking pan.
5. Place a baking pan on the oven rack. Set to air fry at 350 F for 7 minutes.
6. Serve and enjoy.

- **Nutrition Info:** Calories 69 Fat 6.1 g Carbohydrates 1.5 g Sugar 0.5 g Protein 2.5 g Cholesterol 18 mg

282.Baked Apple Slices

Servings: 6
Cooking Time: 30 Minutes
Ingredients:

- 2 apples, peel, core, and slice
- 1 tsp cinnamon
- 2 tbsp butter
- 1/4 cup of sugar
- 1/4 cup brown sugar
- 1/4 tsp salt

Directions:

1. Fit the oven with the rack in position
2. Add cinnamon, sugar, brown sugar, and salt into the zip-lock bag and mix well.
3. Add apple slices into the bag and shake until well coated.
4. Add apple slices into the 9-inch greased baking dish.
5. Set to bake at 350 F for 35 minutes. After 5 minutes place the baking dish in the preheated oven.
6. Serve and enjoy.

- **Nutrition Info:** Calories 128 Fat 4 g Carbohydrates 24.8 g Sugar 21.9 g Protein 0.3 g Cholesterol 10 mg

283.Currant Cookies

Servings: 6
Cooking Time: 15 Minutes
Ingredients:

- ½ cup currants
- ½ cup swerve
- 2 cups almond flour
- ½ cup ghee; melted
- 1 tsp. vanilla extract
- 2 tsp. baking soda

Directions:

1. Take a bowl and mix all the ingredients and whisk well.
2. Spread this on a baking sheet lined with parchment paper, put the pan in the air fryer and cook at 350°F for 30 minutes
3. Cool down; cut into rectangles and serve.

- **Nutrition Info:** Calories: 172; Fat: 5g; Fiber: 2g; Carbs: 3g; Protein: 5g

284.Deep-dish Giant Double Chocolate Chip Cookie

Servings:x
Cooking Time:x
Ingredients:

- 1 large egg
- 1 cup all-purpose flour
- ½ tsp baking powder
- ½ tsp salt
- 1 cup chocolate chip
- ½ cup unsalted butter
- ½ cup light brown sugar
- ½ cup white sugar
- 1 tsp vanilla
- ½ cup chocolate chunks

Directions:

1. Preheat oven to 350°F.
2. Melt butter in oven over low heat.
3. Add sugars and stir well.
4. Incorporate vanilla and egg, and beat quickly to make sure eggs do not cook.
5. Stir in flour, baking soda and salt.
6. Fold in chocolate chips and chunks and spread dough out in oven lightly with a spatula to flatten.
7. Bake for 25 minutes until cookie appears browned on top.

285.Vanilla And Oats Pudding

Servings:x
Cooking Time:x
Ingredients:

- 2 tbsp. custard powder
- 3 tbsp. powdered sugar
- 3 tbsp. unsalted butter
- 2 cups vanilla powder
- 2 cups milk
- 1 cup oats

Directions:

1. Boil the milk and the sugar in a pan and add the custard powder followed by the vanilla powder followed by the oats and stir till you get a thick mixture.
2. Preheat the fryer to 300 Fahrenheit for five minutes. Place the dish in the basket and reduce the temperature to 250 Fahrenheit. Cook for ten minutes and set aside to cool.

286.Nan Khatam

Servings:x
Cooking Time:x
Ingredients:

- 1 tbsp. Unsalted Butter
- 1 tsp. baking powder
- 1 tsp. baking soda
- 1 tsp. cardamom powder
- 1 ½ cup all-purpose flour
- 1 cup Gram flour
- 1 cup +3 tbsp. icing sugar

Directions:

1. Create a crumbly mixture using the ingredients and make small balls of the mixture and flattening them on a prepared baking tray.
2. Preheat the fryer to 300 Fahrenheit for five minutes. Place the baking tray in the basket and reduce the temperature to 250 Fahrenheit. Cook both sides of the ball for five minutes to ensure that they are cooked uniformly. Once the nan khatam has cooled, store them in an airtight container.

287.Sesame Banana Dessert

Servings: 5
Cooking Time: 15 Minutes
Ingredients:

- 1 ½ cups flour
- 5 bananas, sliced
- 1 tsp salt
- 3 tbsp sesame seeds
- 1 cup water
- 2 eggs, beaten
- 1 tsp baking powder
- ½ tbsp sugar

Directions:

1. Preheat on Bake function to 340 F. In a bowl, mix salt, sesame seeds, flour, baking powder, eggs, sugar, and water. Coat sliced bananas with the flour mixture. Place the prepared slices in the Air Fryer basket and fit in the baking tray; cook for 8-10 minutes. Serve chilled.

288.Paprika Potato Chips

Servings:3
Cooking Time: 22 Minutes

Ingredients:

- 2 medium potatoes, preferably Yukon Gold, scrubbed
- Cooking spray
- 2 teaspoons olive oil
- ½ teaspoon garlic granules
- ¼ teaspoon paprika
- ¼ teaspoon plus ⅛ teaspoon sea salt
- ¼ teaspoon freshly ground black pepper
- Ketchup or hot sauce, for serving

Directions:

1. Spritz the air fryer basket with cooking spray.
2. On a flat work surface, cut the potatoes into ¼-inch-thick slices. Transfer the potato slices to a medium bowl, along with the olive oil, garlic granules, paprika, salt, and pepper and toss to coat well. Transfer the potato slices to the basket.
3. Put the air fryer basket on the baking pan and slide into Rack Position 2, select Air Fry, set temperature to 392ºF (200ºC), and set time to 22 minutes.
4. Stir the potato slices twice during the cooking process.
5. When cooking is complete, the potato chips should be tender and nicely browned. Remove from the oven and serve alongside the ketchup for dipping.

289.Garlic Cheese Dip

Servings: 10
Cooking Time: 15 Minutes
Ingredients:

- 1 lb. mozzarella; shredded
- 6 garlic cloves; minced
- 3 tbsp. olive oil
- 1 tbsp. thyme; chopped.
- 1 tsp. rosemary; chopped.
- A pinch of salt and black pepper

Directions:

1. In a pan that fits your air fryer, mix all the ingredients, whisk really well, introduce in the air fryer and cook at 370°F for 10 minutes.
2. Divide into bowls and serve right away.

- **Nutrition Info:** Calories: 184; Fat: 11g; Fiber: 3g; Carbs: 5g; Protein: 7g

290.Buttered Dinner Rolls

Servings: 12
Cooking Time: 30 Minutes
Ingredients:

- 1 cup milk
- 3 cups plain flour
- 7½ tablespoons unsalted butter
- 1 tablespoon coconut oil
- 1 tablespoon olive oil
- 1 teaspoon yeast
- Salt and black pepper, to taste

Directions:

1. Preheat the Air fryer to 360 degree F and grease an Air fryer basket.
2. Put olive oil, milk and coconut oil in a pan and cook for about 3 minutes.
3. Remove from the heat and mix well.
4. Mix together plain flour, yeast, butter, salt and black pepper in a large bowl.
5. Knead well for about 5 minutes until a dough is formed.
6. Cover the dough with a damp cloth and keep aside for about 5 minutes in a warm place.
7. Knead the dough for about 5 minutes again with your hands.
8. Cover the dough with a damp cloth and keep aside for about 30 minutes in a warm place.
9. Divide the dough into 12 equal pieces and roll each into a ball.
10. Arrange 6 balls into the Air fryer basket in a single layer and cook for about 15 minutes.
11. Repeat with the remaining balls and serve warm.

- **Nutrition Info:** Calories: 208, Fat: 10.3g, Carbohydrates: 25g, Sugar: 1g, Protein: 4.1g, Sodium: 73mg

291.Creamy Chicken Dip

Servings: 6
Cooking Time: 20 Minutes
Ingredients:

- 2 cups chicken, cooked and shredded
- 8 oz cream cheese, softened
- 3 tbsp hot sauce
- 1/4 tsp garlic powder
- 3/4 cup sour cream

- 1/4 tsp onion powder

Directions:

1. Fit the oven with the rack in position 2.
2. Add all ingredients in a large bowl and mix until well combined.
3. Transfer mixture in air fryer baking dish.
4. Set to bake at 325 F for 25 minutes. After 5 minutes place the baking dish in the preheated oven.
5. Serve and enjoy.

- **Nutrition Info:** Calories 265 Fat 20.7 g Carbohydrates 2.5 g Sugar 0.3 g Protein 17.4 g Cholesterol 90 mg

292.Zucchini Coconut Bites

Servings: 6
Cooking Time: 10 Minutes

Ingredients:

- 4 zucchini, grated and squeeze out all liquid
- 1 cup shredded coconut
- 1 egg, lightly beaten
- 1 tsp Italian seasoning
- 1/2 cup parmesan cheese, grated

Directions:

1. Fit the oven with the rack in position 2.
2. Add all ingredients into the bowl and mix until well combined.
3. Make small balls from the zucchini mixture and place in the air fryer basket then place the air fryer basket in the baking pan.
4. Place a baking pan on the oven rack. Set to air fry at 400 F for 10 minutes.
5. Serve and enjoy.

- **Nutrition Info:** Calories 105 Fat 7.3 g Carbohydrates 6.8 g Sugar 3.2 g Protein 5.4 g Cholesterol 33 mg

293.Polenta Fries With Chili-lime Mayo

Servings:4
Cooking Time: 28 Minutes

Ingredients:

- Polenta Fries:
- 2 teaspoons vegetable or olive oil
- ¼ teaspoon paprika
- 1 pound (454 g) prepared polenta, cut into 3-inch × ½-inch strips
- Salt and freshly ground black pepper, to taste
- Chili-Lime Mayo:
- ½ cup mayonnaise
- 1 teaspoon chili powder
- 1 teaspoon chopped fresh cilantro
- ¼ teaspoon ground cumin
- Juice of ½ lime
- Salt and freshly ground black pepper, to taste

Directions:

1. Mix the oil and paprika in a bowl. Add the polenta strips and toss until evenly coated. Transfer the polenta strips to the air fryer basket.
2. Put the air fryer basket on the baking pan and slide into Rack Position 2, select Air Fry, set temperature to 400ºF (205ºC), and set time to 28 minutes.
3. Stir the polenta strips halfway through the cooking time.
4. Meanwhile, whisk together all the ingredients for the chili-lime mayo in a small bowl.
5. When cooking is complete, remove the polenta fries from the oven to a plate. Season as desired with salt and pepper. Serve alongside the chili-lime mayo as a dipping sauce.

294.Cardamom Cakes

Servings:x
Cooking Time:x

Ingredients:

- 2 tbsp. butter
- 2 tbsp. sugar
- Muffin cups
- 2 cups All-purpose flour
- 1 ½ cup milk
- 1 tbsp. cardamom powder
- ½ tsp. baking powder
- ½ tsp. baking soda

Directions:

1. Mix the ingredients together and use your Oregano Fingers to get a crumbly mixture.
2. Add the baking soda and the vinegar to the milk and mix continuously. Add this milk to the mixture and create a batter, which you will need to transfer to the muffin cups.

3. Preheat the fryer to 300 Fahrenheit for five minutes. You will need to place the muffin cups in the basket and cover it. Cook the muffins for fifteen minutes and check whether or not the muffins are cooked using a toothpick. Remove the cups and serve hot.

295.Fruity Oreo Muffins

Servings: 6
Cooking Time: 10 Minutes
Ingredients:

- 1 cup milk
- 1 pack Oreo biscuits, crushed
- ¾ teaspoon baking powder
- 1 banana, peeled and chopped
- 1 apple, peeled, cored and chopped
- 1 teaspoon cocoa powder
- 1 teaspoon honey
- 1 teaspoon fresh lemon juice
- A pinch of ground cinnamon

Directions:

1. Preheat the Air fryer to 320 degree F and grease 6 muffin cups lightly.
2. Mix milk, biscuits, cocoa powder, baking soda, and baking powder in a bowl until well combined.
3. Transfer the mixture into the muffin cups and cook for about 10 minutes.
4. Remove from the Air fryer and invert the muffin cups onto a wire rack to cool.
5. Meanwhile, mix the banana, apple, honey, lemon juice, and cinnamon in another bowl.
6. Scoop some portion of muffins from the center and fill with fruit mixture to serve.

- **Nutrition Info:** Calories: 182, Fat: 3.1g, Carbohydrates: 31.4g, Sugar: 19.5g, Protein: 3.1g, Sodium: 196mg

296.Crunchy Chickpeas

Servings:4
Cooking Time: 18 Minutes
Ingredients:

- ½ teaspoon chili powder
- ½ teaspoon ground cumin
- ¼ teaspoon cayenne pepper
- ¼ teaspoon salt
- 1 (19-ounce / 539-g) can chickpeas, drained and rinsed
- Cooking spray

Directions:

1. Lina the air fryer basket with parchment paper and lightly spritz with cooking spray.
2. Mix the chili powder, cumin, cayenne pepper, and salt in a small bowl.
3. Place the chickpeas in a medium bowl and lightly mist with cooking spray.
4. Add the spice mixture to the chickpeas and toss until evenly coated. Transfer the chickpeas to the parchment.
5. Put the air fryer basket on the baking pan and slide into Rack Position 2, select Air Fry, set temperature to 390ºF (199ºC), and set time to 18 minutes.
6. Stir the chickpeas twice during cooking.
7. When cooking is complete, the chickpeas should be crunchy. Remove from the oven and let the chickpeas cool for 5 minutes before serving.

297.Spicy And Sweet Roasted Nuts

Servings: 4 Cups
Cooking Time: 15 Minutes
Ingredients:

- 1 pound (454 g) walnut halves and pieces
- ½ cup granulated sugar
- 3 tablespoons vegetable oil
- 1 teaspoon cayenne pepper
- ½ teaspoon fine salt

Directions:

1. Soak the walnuts in a large bowl with boiling water for a minute or two. Drain the walnuts. Stir in the sugar, oil and cayenne pepper to coat well. Spread the walnuts in a single layer in the baking pan.
2. Slide the baking pan into Rack Position 2, select Roast, set temperature to 325ºF (163ºC) and set time to 15 minutes.
3. After 7 or 8 minutes, remove from the oven. Stir the nuts. Return the pan to the oven and continue cooking, check frequently.
4. When cooking is complete, the walnuts should be dark golden brown. Remove from the oven. Sprinkle the nuts with the salt and let cool. Serve warm.

298.Apple Treat With Raisins

Servings:4
Cooking Time: 15 Minutes
Ingredients:

- 4 apples, cored
- 1 ½ oz almonds
- ¾ oz raisins
- 2 tbsp sugar

Directions:

1. Preheat on Bake function to 360 F. In a bowl, mix sugar, almonds, and raisins and blend the mixture using a hand mixer. Fill cored apples with the almond mixture. Place the prepared apples in the basket and press Start. Bake for 10 minutes. Serve with powdered sugar.

299.Strawberry And Rhubarb Crumble

Servings:6
Cooking Time: 12 To 17 Minutes
Ingredients:

- 1½ cups sliced fresh strawberries
- $^{1}/_{3}$ cup sugar
- ¾ cup sliced rhubarb
- $^{2}/_{3}$ cup quick-cooking oatmeal
- ¼ cup packed brown sugar
- ½ cup whole-wheat pastry flour
- ½ teaspoon ground cinnamon
- 3 tablespoons unsalted butter, melted

Directions:

1. Place the strawberries, sugar, and rhubarb in the baking pan and toss to coat.
2. Combine the oatmeal, brown sugar, pastry flour, and cinnamon in a medium bowl.
3. Add the melted butter to the oatmeal mixture and stir until crumbly. Sprinkle this generously on top of the strawberries and rhubarb.
4. Slide the baking pan into Rack Position 1, select Convection Bake, set temperature to 370ºF (188ºC), and set the time to 12 minutes.
5. Bake until the fruit is bubbly and the topping is golden brown. Continue cooking for an additional 2 to 5 minutes if needed.
6. When cooking is complete, remove from the oven and serve warm.

300.Roasted Veggie Bowl

Servings: 2
Cooking Time: 35 Minutes
Ingredients:

- ¼ medium white onion; peeled.and sliced ¼-inch thick
- ½ medium green bell pepper; seeded and sliced ¼-inch thick
- 1 cup broccoli florets
- 1 cup quartered Brussels sprouts
- ½ cup cauliflower florets
- 1 tbsp. coconut oil
- ½ tsp. garlic powder.
- ½ tsp. cumin
- 2 tsp. chili powder

Directions:

1. Toss all ingredients together in a large bowl until vegetables are fully coated with oil and seasoning. Pour vegetables into the air fryer basket.
2. Adjust the temperature to 360 Degrees F and set the timer for 15 minutes. Shake two- or three-times during cooking. Serve warm.

- **Nutrition Info:** Calories: 121; Protein: 4.3g; Fiber: 5.2g; Fat: 7.1g; Carbs: 13.1g

Milton Keynes UK
Ingram Content Group UK Ltd.
UKHW031813110124
435868UK00007B/586